the
food
medic

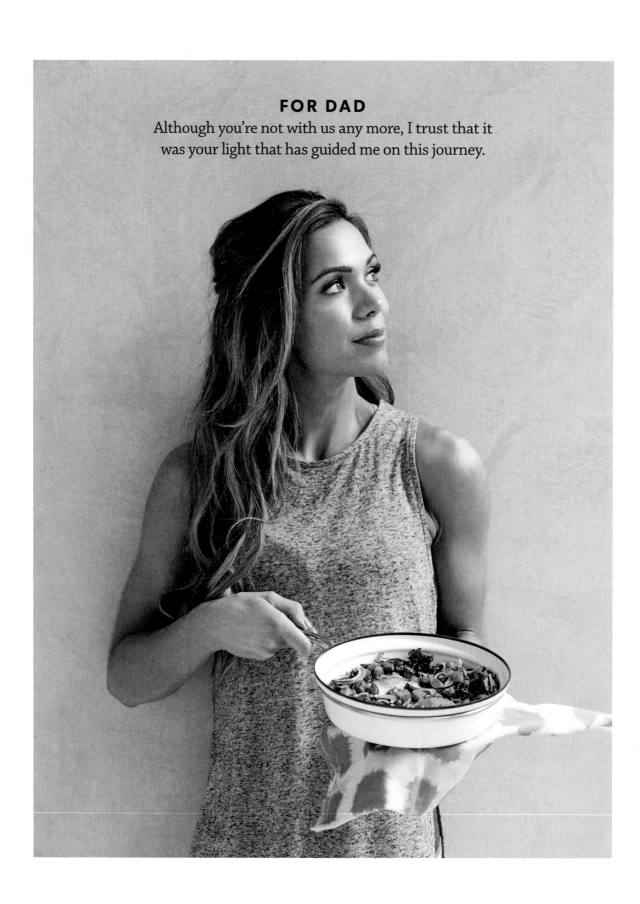

FOR DAD

Although you're not with us any more, I trust that it was your light that has guided me on this journey.

out from underneath me. Everything I knew – my stability, my foundations – just collapsed. Initially I had no idea how profoundly I had been affected – I carried on working hard and going to school. I tried to remain focused and disciplined, not least because I didn't want to give my mum anything else to worry about. But soon things started to crumble and I began to worry now that Dad wasn't there to lean on.

I became anxious, particularly about money and how Mum would cope paying for my school, how we would pay the bills. The way my dad died also made me question health and well-being – could we have spotted something or were there obvious signs that he wasn't well and we just didn't know what to look for? It took me a long time to accept that someone so obviously healthy could simply die with no warning, doing something as mundane as eating dinner.

I think that was the point at which the seed was sown for me wanting to become a doctor and understand how food affected health – somewhere in the back of my mind was the idea that, if I had as much medical knowledge as it was possible to have, it could help me protect myself and the people I loved in a way I hadn't been able to do for Dad. I always worked hard at school so I decided to throw myself into studying medicine with everything I had. But then I stopped being able to eat.

Life had been changed forever and it wasn't that I stopped eating because I feared food or because I wanted control – I genuinely just felt too sad to put food in my mouth and chew it and I stopped looking at it as a positive and life-giving thing. It became another chore that I couldn't face. Our house was as noisy and full as it had ever been, particularly when Mum decided to take in a foster child, and, outwardly, I appeared to be coping fine. But I

was disappearing both mentally and physically, and I think I became fixated on mortality. I had a Saturday job in the small village pharmacy and I knew the name of every drug on the shelf – I also knew the name of every customer, many of whom were very elderly, and I knew that if they didn't come in and collect their prescription that probably meant they were dead.

The only way I could describe how I felt was as being too sad for life – too sad to eat or to contemplate moving forward with life after my dad's death. I was paralysed by grief. My mum took me to my GP and I went willingly – my dad dying so suddenly had shown me that death could happen any time to anyone and I was terrified that my body would give up. I was desperate to make things right, but I just couldn't seem to do what I needed to. I didn't know how or what to eat to make me feel better.

I was so driven at school because all I wanted was to do well, to get my grades and become a doctor, and I didn't want anything to get in the way of that. There isn't a name for someone who is so crippled by loss that the very act of thinking about taking pleasure in food is impossible. I can see now that I was suffering from depression. My GP was very supportive and referred me for counselling, which was a bit of a disaster: because I was so thin, they were adamant that I was anorexic and tried to have me hospitalised on a drip. That was the turning point really – I knew that wasn't what was wrong with me and I vowed that I would make myself better without medical intervention. There isn't always a pill for every ill. It was more that my mind couldn't process all the changes and the deep sense of heartbreak I felt at losing my dad. I knew I had to find a way to feed my body as that would help my mind.

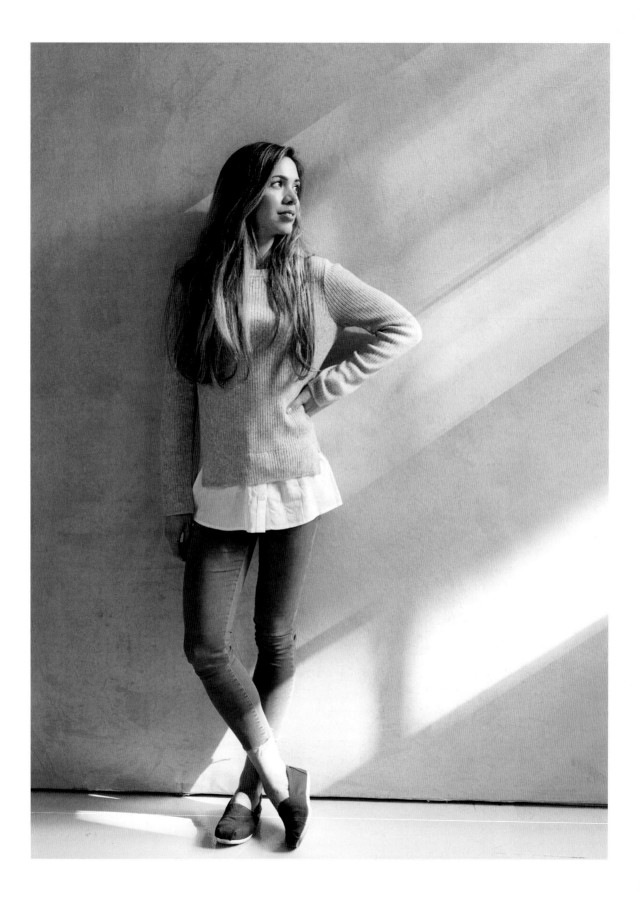

This isn't a book with a collection of recipes that will just help shift a few stubborn pounds before or after a holiday; it is about health, confidence, happiness and feeling great. We all feel our best when we are free of illness, full of energy and at a healthy weight. I am going to show you how to maximise your health through nutrition and teach you, step-by-step, healthy eating habits for life so you will never have to diet again.

In my recipes, and in my own life, I try to use the most natural, unrefined and unprocessed, whole-food ingredients. The purity of such foods not only nourishes your body physically, but emotionally and mentally. I want to help banish the myths around healthy eating and diets, and instead help to promote this type of eating as a way of life.

HOW IT ALL BEGAN

Food has always been a huge part of my life. Everyone has their own individual relationship with food – mine was wonderfully uncomplicated until I was fourteen years old and my father died suddenly.

Before then, you could say that I celebrated food on a daily basis. My mum always says that I enjoyed every single meal from as early as she can remember – her best memories are of me kneeling at the dining table, talking to everyone as they ate their food, discussing what was on the plate, how it tasted and if they liked it. In fact, the childhood story goes that I used to eat dinner on a Saturday and spend the whole time discussing what we would have for dessert after Sunday lunch.

We were brought up to appreciate and respect 'real' food – my mum always bought things fresh and, if my friends came round and wanted chips, my mum would make them from scratch and wrap them up in newspaper so they felt like they were from the chip shop. Every week we would go to the library and borrow three books each, and I would always take out one recipe book and two Roald Dahls. I would

sit for hours in the library browsing through recipes and imagining how they would taste and if I could persuade my mum to make them.

I remember very clearly that each meal always had to look nice and be full of colour, even when I was really young and I would hover in the kitchen with my hand in every pot, 'helping'. I adored colourful food and I would eat anything, even if it was raw and unpeeled and just in its natural state. I was healthy and happy and loved life.

Then my father died and everything was turned upside down. Even though he was older than my mum, he was full of life before he suffered a stroke at the dining table in front of the whole family. We were sitting down to a family meal, just like we always did and everything imploded. It seemed that even though he'd recently been diagnosed with high blood pressure, overhauled his diet and started exercising, the damage had already been done. He was taken to hospital and several days later he died there. His death changed my life in every way – it is hard to explain really except that I felt like the rug had been pulled right

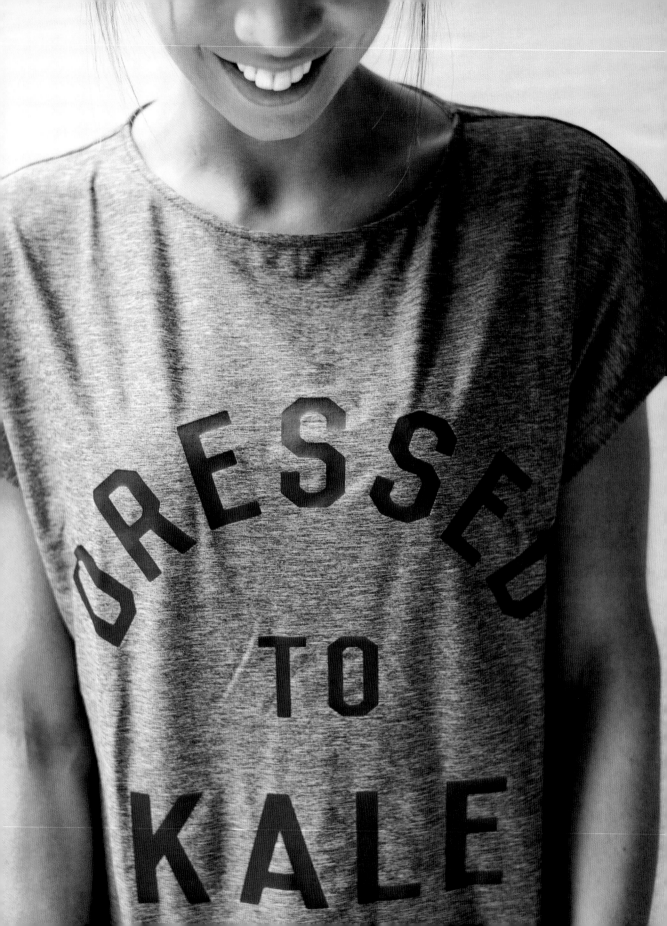

FOREWORD

With the mass of 'clean eating', 'wellness' and 'diet' books on the market today, you may be rolling your eyes and wondering how this book is any different to the rest of them?

- This book is different.
- There's nothing out there like it.
- This book combines medicine, health, nutrition and fitness.

As a qualified doctor, personal trainer and a self-confessed health foodie, this book combines my areas of expertise to offer you a full-body guide to health and well-being.

This book isn't about quick fixes, detoxes, or diet myths. It's about good quality, scientifically backed-up advice from a straight-talking doctor, but also from someone who has experienced first-hand how food can drastically impact your health.

I WANT THIS BOOK TO:
- help you rethink your relationship with food
- teach you the basics of good nutrition
- allow you to create your own healthy pattern of eating so that you never have to diet again
- encourage you to cook simple, healthy dishes from scratch
- help you fall in love with your body with easy-to-follow, tailor-made workouts
- help you maximise your health and prevent disease, through food

This book is about the celebration of real food, good habits and an understanding of how the food we put into our bodies has consequences for every aspect of our physical and mental well-being.

Hazel xx

CONTENTS

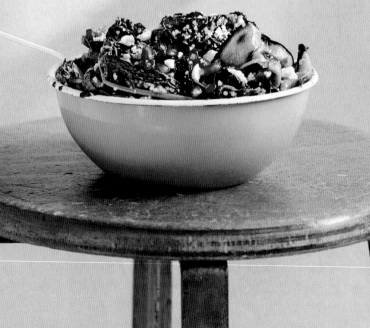

First published in Great Britain in 2017 by Yellow Kite
An imprint of Hodder & Stoughton
An Hachette UK company
1
Copyright © Dr Hazel Wallace 2017

Photography: Susan Bell
Art direction and design: Nikki Dupin
Food styling: Frankie Unsworth
Props and styling: Olivia Wardle
Emoji art on page 35 supplied by EmojiOne

A CIP catalogue record for this title is available from the British Library

Hardback ISBN 978 1 473 65053 4
Ebook ISBN 978 1 473 65052 7

The advice herein is not intended to replace the services of trained health and fitness professionals,
or be a substitute for medical advice. You are advised to consult with your health care professional
with regards to matters relating to your health, and in particular regarding matters that may
require diagnosis or medical attention.

Printed and bound in Germany by Mohn Media
Hodder & Stoughton policy is to use papers that are natural, renewable and recyclable products and made from
wood grown in sustainable forests. The logging and manufacturing processes are expected to conform to the
environmental regulations of the country of origin.

Hodder & Stoughton Ltd
Carmelite House
50 Victoria Embankment
London EC4Y 0DZ

www.yellowkitebooks.co.uk
www.hodder.co.uk

the
food
medic

RECIPES + FITNESS FOR A
HEALTHIER, HAPPIER YOU

DR HAZEL WALLACE

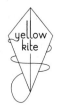

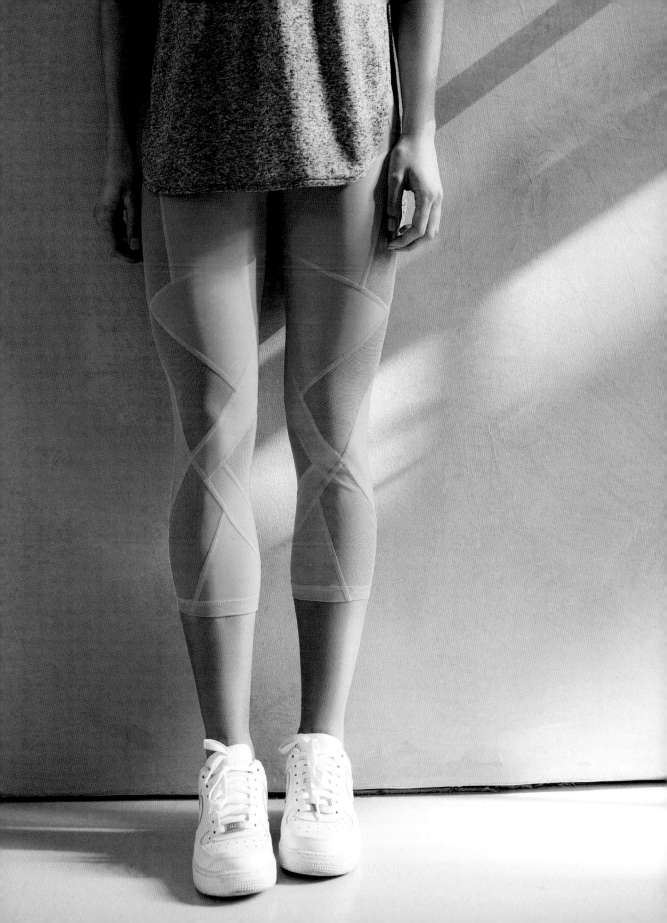

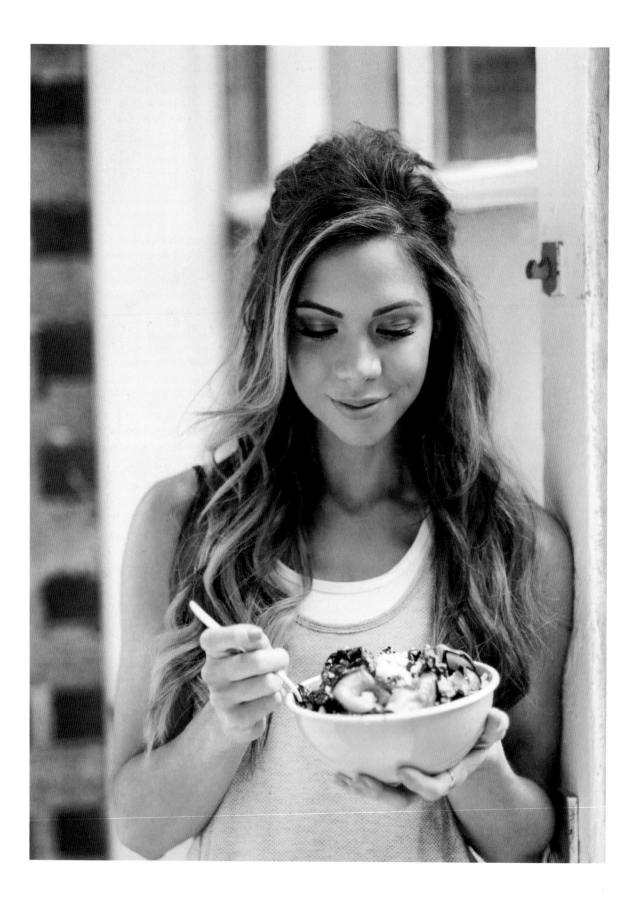

I asked to be referred to a dietician, one of the best decisions I ever made. Going to see her turned my life around and gave me a whole new perspective on food and nourishment, and I never looked back. She gave me precise weekly targets, lists of foods and calorie intake goals to help strengthen me up. Mum always says that the turning point for her was when I asked to go to McDonald's for a milkshake; that's when she knew I was going to be OK. The dietician helped me rediscover my joy around food, so even when the goal was to bulk up, I never lost sight of the fact that food always had to look and taste good.

I think working with the dietician was the moment I discovered a deep-rooted belief in nourishing the mind as well as the body. Week by week I watched the weight on the scales creep up; I felt my body getting stronger and becoming more feminine, but I also felt my mind rebooting and coming back to life. Initially I was scared to exercise, in case I would slow down my progress back to a healthy weight but my dietician and GP encouraged me. I started with walks in the evening, swimming on the weekends, and joined a yoga class at the local hotel – and even managed to drag my mum along with me. Although it was a very low-intensity activity, it made me feel amazing and it showed me how strong my body was becoming. Physical exercise became another core strand of recovery for me and remains a vital part of my daily routine.

I was back to a healthy weight, and back to my usual happy self, just in time for my final exams at secondary school. Unfortunately it was too little too late, and the eighteen months I had spent between depression and my recovery meant my grades at school had slipped. When my leaving certificate results came out, my heart sank as I stared down at the piece of paper with a 'B' beside all nine

subjects I had taken. I didn't get an offer to study medicine at the schools I had applied for in Ireland, but I did get an offer to study a bachelor's degree in Medical Sciences in Wales. I wasn't ready to give up my dream of becoming a doctor so at the age of eighteen I packed my bags and left for Pontypridd in South Wales.

This was the next big chapter of my life, and a far cry from the previous one. It was my first time living away from home, never mind living in a new country, and my first year at university. I was ready to fully embrace uni life – the socials, the all-nighters, the 3 a.m. trips to the takeaway! The student lifestyle, coupled with the stress of exams and the pressure to get into medical school, made me develop an unhealthy relationship with food. When I was busy revising for exams or working towards an assignment deadline, I would eat whatever comfort food I could get my hands on. I was living on bags of Doritos, bowls of Frosties and microwaveable meals. From this, I would bounce to extremes of trying to follow 'healthy' diets, which included cereal bars, sweetened yogurts, and 'slimming' meals and snacks. I was consuming an excessive amount of sugar, and completely under-eating in terms of my protein, fats and calories. Although I was still slim, I had gone from a size 6 to a size 10–12 in a couple of months. I was lethargic, I had dry skin and hair, and most of all, I completely lacked body confidence.

When I flew back home for Easter break in my first year of uni, I had my wake-up call. I remember standing in my kitchen and one of my mother's friends commented on how much I had 'filled' out. It didn't really affect me too much at the time, and I shrugged the comment off. During the same week I went out with my old school friends and the day after, when I was going through the photos from our night out, the penny dropped. I could hardly recognise myself because of how bloated I looked. I was clearly in denial and had tried to squeeze into a size 8 skirt and top, which was much too small for me. That day I broke down and promised myself that I would never let myself feel that uncomfortable and ashamed of my body again. I flew back to Wales for a six-week revision period before my exams and decided to join the gym to keep me motivated and energised while I was studying. Alongside my daily gym regime, I began to do some research into nutrition and tweak my diet. I started to cook meals from scratch, try new foods, and experiment with different ingredients. Something inside me changed and my passion for cooking was reignited.

I developed recipes for myself in my student kitchen. I only had a student budget to work with, little kitchen space and not much time so I learnt to cook quick, inexpensive, healthy meals with what I could afford. I decided to take photographs of my meals and track my physical progress using Instagram. I posted anonymously to start with as my intention was to use it as my own personal diary to health. My followers built up quickly as more and more people became interested in my recipes, workouts and, I guess, my story. I've since developed a huge network of support across social media and it has encouraged me to accumulate all of my experience, knowledge and passion to write this book. I am the first of a new generation of doctors who see the importance of nutrition as the cornerstone to healthcare.

NUTRITION IN MEDICAL SCHOOL

Nutrition is not a subject that is heavily focused on, or even taught, at medical school in the UK and across the world. It's surprising given that most healthcare systems, including the NHS, aim to focus as much on promoting wellness as they do treating and managing disease.

Of course as medical students we learnt about the anatomy and physiology of the digestive system and metabolism of nutrients in the body, but the practical application of nutrition, and the translation from textbook to clinical practice, is something that we don't learn in medical school.

As part of my undergraduate bachelor's degree in Medical Sciences, I studied a module in human nutrition which gave me a solid foundation on the basics of nutrition. However, despite being able to tell you the blood supply to the small bowel, I wouldn't have been able to tell you practical things like the minimum amount of protein we need each day, or what a balanced meal should be made up of. So with my basic understanding of nutrition and the ability to read scientific papers and journals, I set out on my own and decided to educate myself on this topic – and so The Food Medic was born.

Although nutrition is just one pillar of the foundation to good public health, it massively contributes to the prevention of some of the most common killers: heart disease, stroke and cancer. I personally feel that it is something that the medical profession overlooks and under-utilises as a means of reducing the rates of such lifestyle-related diseases.

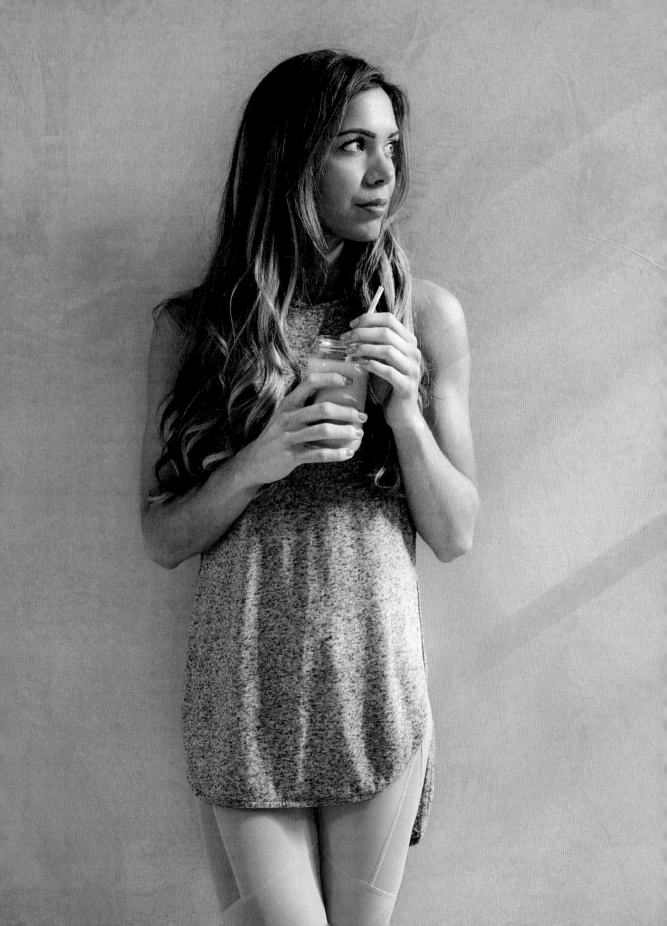

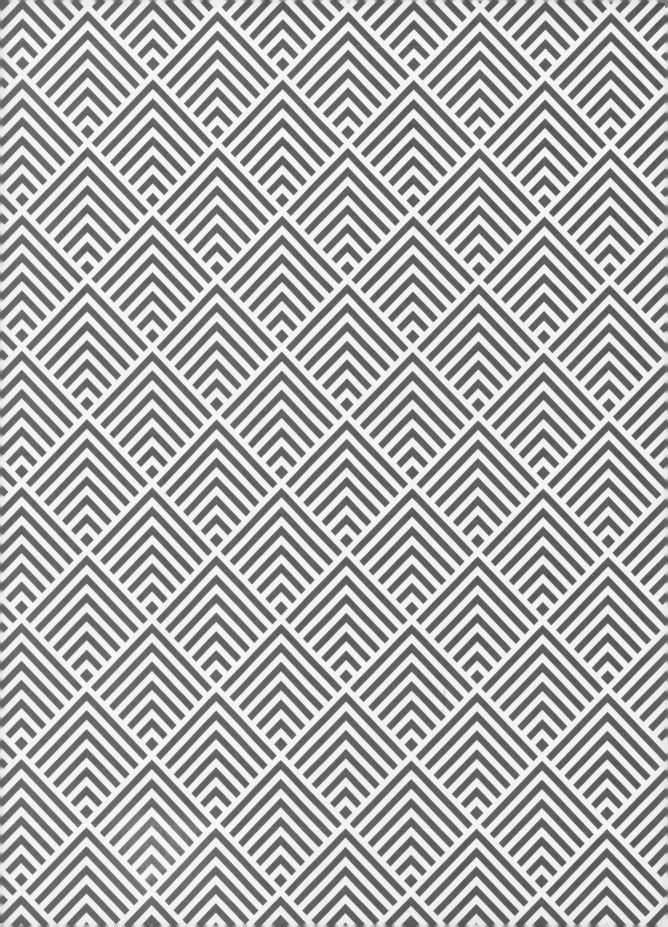

NUTRITION

—

THE BASICS

Q: Have you ever gone on a diet, maybe lost a few pounds, only to put it back on again?

A: Yep, I've been there too.

Q: Have you ever tried a diet that doesn't involve some form of restriction, whether it's sugar, fats, bread or another type of 'bad' food?

A: Nope? Me neither.

When I was underweight, my focus was on eating whatever calorie-rich foods I could get my hands on. I wasn't concerned about the nutritional content of the food, I just knew that the more calories I could eat in a day, the faster I would put on weight. It became a numbers game for me, and the number of calories consumed and pounds gained were my targets. I had weekly weigh-ins with my dietician and I would stand on the scales and close my eyes, praying the number would be higher than the previous week. I wanted nothing more than to be a healthy weight again and have my life back.

A couple of years down the line, when I moved away to university and gained the dreaded 'freshers' fifteen'*, it was only natural for me to think in numbers again – if increasing calories made me gain weight, then I should restrict my calories in order to lose weight. It seemed logical, but despite restricting my food intake I wasn't making much progress.

I fell into the trap that many others do and tried every diet in the book: a cereal diet, a fruit-only diet, a juice diet, and even meal replacement shakes. I cringe just thinking about how naive I was, but I was so unhappy and uncomfortable that I was desperate to try anything that worked. The thing is – none of them worked.

'Hangry'** and frustrated with my lack of results I decided to take matters into my own hands and do what I do best – research. I started to educate myself on the basics of nutrition and study the different dietary approaches, and the evidence for each. I soon realised that I was eating the completely wrong type of food – if you can call it food.

What I perceived as 'healthy' were foods labelled 'low cal', 'low fat' or 'diet'. After doing some research, I took a closer look and realised my diet was actually far from healthy and full of processed foods which were high in sugar, low in protein and lacking healthy fats.

That's when the penny dropped. Could I really follow a diet which would allow me to eat more, lose weight and improve my health? And was the solution really as simple as ditching my 'low-cal' snacks for real food? The answer is yes, it really is that simple. I was focusing on what I should be cutting out, rather than what I should be including – lean protein, wholesome carbohydrates and healthy fats.

I'll put my hands up now and admit that it wasn't easy completely transforming my diet, and unfortunately it didn't happen overnight. Initially I missed the convenience of popping to the takeaway after a long day of uni, or pouring myself a bowl of cereal before dashing out the door at 6 a.m. Thankfully, my determination to succeed was much greater than my laziness or lack of will. I cleared out my fridge and cupboards of any junk and processed foods, and restocked them with whole foods like fresh fruit, vegetables, nuts, seeds, lean meats and fish. I started to cook my meals from scratch (which involved lots of trial and error) and prep my lunches the night before.

Alongside my new diet, I joined a gym and started resistance-based training for the first time in my life. My strength was poor – I could barely lift the lightest weights in the gym. I also felt totally clueless trying to work out how each machine worked. However, I stuck to my training programme and got up to go to the gym before the library every day.

I soon noticed that I had more energy in the mornings, my skin improved, my eyes were brighter, my clothes fitted better and my tummy felt flatter. I fell back in love with cooking and experimenting with new foods. I had no idea that healthy foods could be this delicious or satisfying. It was then that I started to view food as medicine. I realised food wasn't the enemy and, chosen well, it has the potential to improve health and keep illness at bay.

As the saying goes, knowledge is power, and in order to kickstart and maintain a healthy diet and lifestyle, it is important to understand the basics of good nutrition. A healthy diet needs to be flexible and sustainable. No one wants to eat the same salad for lunch every day or stress about not having the five cashew nuts at 11 a.m. that their diet outlined. It can be overwhelming to try to stick to a diet plan and, if you fall off the bespoke diet wagon, it can lead to feelings of guilt and failure. Before I had an understanding of nutrition, I thought there was only one right way of doing things. If I didn't eat that tuna and jacket potato for lunch that was written in my diet plan, then I would undo all my good work and pile back on the pounds. I know, it's totally illogical but I felt like if I didn't stick to my plan 100 per cent of the time, then I was failing. What made the process easier for me is that I understood why I needed to eat this way. I can assemble a healthy meal without thinking about it now. Every meal is an opportunity to nourish our body. I look down at my plate now and see the protein

---

the fifteen pounds freshers traditionally put on in their first year

** hungry and angry*

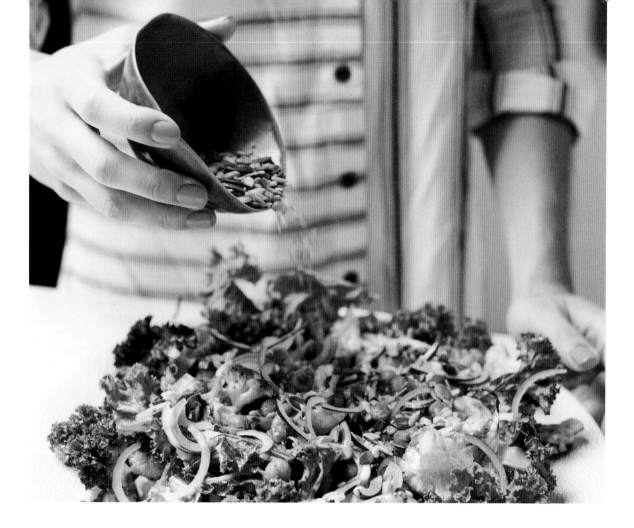

that my body needs to build and repair my muscles, the carbohydrates that give my body energy, and the healthy fats that feed my brain and help me to absorb vitamins and minerals.

I'm not going to give you a strict six-week diet plan, and then leave you on your own to try to keep it up and maintain a healthy diet once the programme is finished. My goal is to set you up for LIFE, not just six weeks. I want to empower you with the right tools to create mindful food choices every day. There are no fads, tricks or gimmicks in this book. The key to changing your lifestyle in order to look better and feel better is stripping your diet back to the basics so you know

exactly what you're fuelling your body with. By understanding how the food you eat impacts on your health, it allows you to make the right choices so that you can transform yourself into a healthier, slimmer and more energetic version of you.

I'm offering you this advice not only as a qualified doctor or a personal trainer, but as a girl who has walked in your shoes. I know first-hand how food can affect both your physical and your mental health. My journey to health has not been easy but deep down I am grateful to have the insight that I do, so that I can pass on my knowledge. Food really is thy medicine.

NUTRIENTS – FOOD IS FUEL BUT SO MUCH MORE

Food is made up of nutrients, which we can mostly break down into macronutrients and micronutrients. The term 'macro' means we require these nutrients in large amounts, and 'micro' in small amounts. Macronutrients (*carbohydrates, proteins and fats*) and micronutrients (*vitamins and minerals*) significantly influence energy levels, our performance, our recovery from exercise, chronic disease progression, body composition and much more.

These nutrients provide energy for the body, in the form of calories.

While each of these macronutrients provides calories, the amount of calories that each one provides varies.

CARBOHYDRATE provides 4 calories per g.

PROTEIN provides 4 calories per g.

FAT provides 9 calories per g.

ALCOHOL provides 7 calories per g.

So it's true that food is fuel, but it's also so much more. Food also contains micronutrients, like vitamins and minerals, and a few other powerful nutrients, such as phytochemicals, antioxidants and even water. Unlike macronutrients, these nutrients do not provide energy, but are essential for normal growth, repair and daily functioning of the body.

MACRONUTRIENTS

PROTEIN

WHY DO WE NEED IT?

Protein is vital for building and repairing muscle tissue. Without protein in the diet the body cannot fully recover from activities, such as lifting weights or running. However, protein is not just important for those hitting the gym and looking to build muscle.

PROTEIN IS ALSO ESSENTIAL FOR:

- **Strong hair, skin and nails** – collagen is a very important protein that can be found throughout the body, from our skin, bones and muscles right down to our tiny blood vessels. The protein keratin is responsible for strong hair and nails. Many expensive hair treatments use this protein in their products to strengthen damaged hair.

- **A strong immune system** – some proteins, known as antibodies, help keep us healthy by defending against disease-causing bacteria and viruses.

- **Important enzymes** – enzymes are types of proteins that speed up reactions in the body, such as the chemical breakdown of food during digestion. Lactase is an enzyme that breaks down lactose, the sugar in milk and dairy, and people who lack this enzyme can't tolerate dairy and suffer from symptoms like bloating of the stomach, abdominal cramps, flatulence, nausea and diarrhoea.

- **The formation of hormones** – insulin, the hormone which regulates our blood sugar levels, is made of protein. Without insulin, we can't use the glucose from the food we eat for energy. People with type 1 diabetes can't produce insulin very well and need to inject themselves with it every day to allow their body to handle glucose appropriately and avoid the complications from high blood sugar, such as eye, kidney, and nerve disease.

- **Back-up fuel** – although carbohydrates and fats are primarily used as our choice fuel sources, protein can be called upon when energy reserves are low, such as during endurance events or periods of fasting.

- **To build and repair muscle** – a large component of muscle tissue is protein so it is important that we get enough through our diet to build, repair and maintain muscle tissue.

- If that wasn't convincing enough, high-protein foods require more energy to digest and metabolise, which means you actually burn more calories processing them. Protein is also very satiating, so it helps to keep you feeling fuller for longer. This means we are less likely to over-indulge on fats or carbohydrates, and actually eat less overall – which is great for anyone watching their waistline.

WHAT IS PROTEIN MADE OF?

Protein is made up of units known as amino acids. There are around twenty-two amino acids in total, and foods high in protein contain different combinations of these. Each amino acid is like a letter of the alphabet and, just as we combine different letters to make different words, different combinations of amino acids make different proteins. So although we only have very few amino acids, they can join together to form large chains.

Most amino acids can be made by our body, but there are nine that we can't make ourselves and so we must get them from food. We call these amino acids 'essential'.

Don't panic, we don't need every essential amino acid in every meal we eat. However, in order to reap the rewards that protein has to offer, we need a sufficient amount of each amino acid every day. Foods that have all nine essential amino acids are called 'complete proteins'. I try to include a complete source of protein with every meal to make sure that I'm doing my very best to support muscle-building and repair. Complete sources of protein are largely animal-based proteins, but plant-based foods, such as quinoa, buckwheat, hemp and chia seeds, contain all the essential amino acids too.

Incomplete proteins are – yes, you guessed it – called incomplete because they don't contain all nine essential amino acids. Essentially, they contain some protein, but they aren't the richest sources of protein. In order to make sure we are getting the whole set of amino acids that we need, we can combine different sources of protein. For example, legumes (beans, peas and lentils) contain an essential amino acid called lysine, which is low in many grains, and grains have the amino acids legumes are generally not very rich in. So by mixing them together in a meal, we can maximise the protein content. If I'm having a meat-free meal, I make sure to combine different grains, legumes, and vegetables so I'm not missing out on my essential amino acids.

Here are some of my favourite ways to combine different incomplete protein sources to make a more protein-rich meal:

LENTIL CURRY & BROWN RICE	PEANUT BUTTER & RYE TOAST	HUMMUS & SEEDED CRACKERS

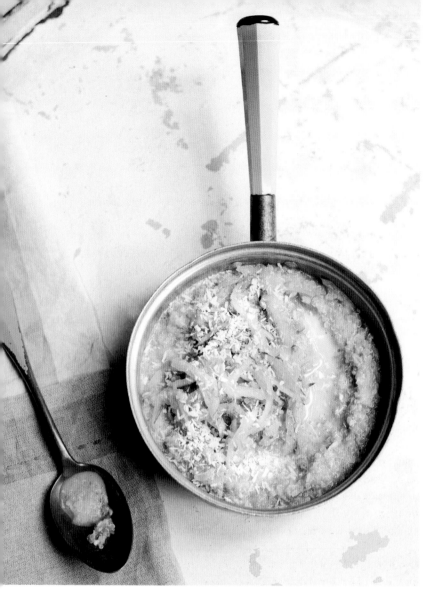

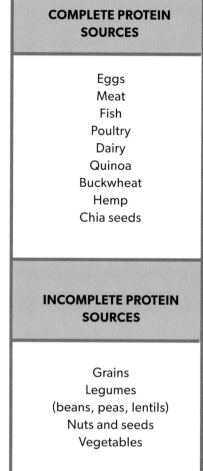

COMPLETE PROTEIN SOURCES
Eggs
Meat
Fish
Poultry
Dairy
Quinoa
Buckwheat
Hemp
Chia seeds

INCOMPLETE PROTEIN SOURCES
Grains
Legumes (beans, peas, lentils)
Nuts and seeds
Vegetables

SO HOW MUCH PROTEIN SHOULD WE BE CONSUMING?

One of the biggest (if not the biggest) changes I made when I transformed my diet was actively including good quality protein in all my meals. Looking back, I would often go a full day without eating much protein at all. It's quite astonishing when you compare my diet then to my diet now. I completely underestimated the importance of protein and often skipped it in order to cut calories. I viewed it as something which was non-essential to my diet, and only useful for body-builders and athletes. Oh, how I could not have been more wrong. Not only do high-protein diets help build and repair muscle, they can also curb hunger, enhance satiety and promote weight loss.

	DIET BEFORE	DIET AFTER
BREAKFAST	Frosties and skimmed milk	Protein oats
LUNCH	Fruit salad, tub of 'low-cal' sweetened yogurt	Chicken and vegetables
DINNER	Baked potato, cheese and beans	Salmon fillet, sweet potato mash, salad
SNACKS	Packet of crisps, cereal bar, jelly sweets	Dark chocolate, apple and almond butter
PROTEIN* TOTAL	**44g**	**100g**

* Estimation only

The British Nutrition Foundation recommends that the average adult consume, 0.75g of protein per kg of body weight per day. However, our protein requirements increase with factors, such as age, pregnancy and breastfeeding, illness, and activity levels. Anyone who works out regularly through resistance training, and other forms of exercise, should increase their protein intake in the range of 1.2–1.7g per kg of body weight per day. This is important to not only build muscle tissue, but to help with recovery and prevent muscle breakdown. If our diet is severely lacking in protein, especially essential amino acids, the body breaks down its richest source of protein – muscle – to access them. So if you're doing sit-ups every day to get washboard abs, you're not going to get that defined six-pack without enough protein in your diet.

WHAT HAPPENS IF I DON'T HAVE ENOUGH PROTEIN?

Severe protein malnutrition is pretty rare in the developed world, but consistently under-eating protein every day can impact health and performance. The signs and symptoms may be mild and often go unnoticed. For example, we know protein is essential for building muscle so if you aren't getting enough of it, you may feel weak and take longer to recover after exercise. Our immune system can also suffer if it doesn't have enough protein to make antibodies, our defence cells, to protect us against colds and flu. Protein isn't just important for strong muscles and strong immune systems, but also strong hair and nails. If you are not consuming enough protein in your diet, your hair is likely to become dry and brittle and your nails may break more easily.

CARBOHYDRATES

'No carbs before Marbs' . . .
'No carbs after six' . . .
'No pizza before Ibiza'

When it comes to dropping fat fast, the first thing we seem to cut from our diet is carbohydrates. Low carb diets became popular with the Atkins craze in the 1990s and many people now associate carbohydrates with weight gain.

The reason many lose weight on a low-carb diet has nothing to do with the fact that carbs are inherently bad for you, it's more to do with the dramatic calorie deficit you put yourself in. If carbs make up a large chunk of your diet and you stop eating them, you'll be consuming considerably fewer total calories. Carbohydrates are found in pretty much everything – from fruit and vegetables, to grains and legumes, but also processed foods, such as sweets and chocolate.

The problem is not eating carbs, but rather, not eating the right carbs. We tend to lump all carbohydrates in the same category, when really they all act very differently in our body. Some are more nutritionally dense than others, such as blueberries and spinach; some are digested slower, such as oats and brown rice, and therefore have less of an impact on our blood sugar levels; and some are packed full of fibre, like carrots, squash and broccoli. However, refined sugar, like that in sweets and chocolate, lacks fibre so it doesn't fill

you up (and leaves you constipated), causes fluctuations in blood sugar leaving you full of energy one minute and sleeping at your desk the next, and is generally full of added chemicals, flavours and preservatives, which I'm not even going to start to list or try to pronounce.

Take a bowl of sugary cereal, which is packed full of refined carbohydrates, and compare it to a bowl of porridge oats. I know I could easily work my way through two or three bowls of cereal without feeling full and that I will feel tired immediately afterwards, not to mention hungry one or two hours later. However, with my bowl of porridge oats, I always feel full and satisfied, with hours of energy to power through until lunch. So let's take a closer look at the different types of carbohydrates and where we can find the best sources to include in our diet.

NOT ALL CARBOHYDRATES ARE CREATED EQUAL

First, let's talk about how our body breaks down and uses carbohydrates.

Carbohydrates are the main source of energy in the body, but in order to use that energy, all carbohydrates need to first be broken down to their simplest form – glucose. Glucose provides fuel for every cell in your body, particularly your brain and nerve cells. The brain, despite only accounting for 2 per cent of our entire body weight, uses 20 per cent of the glucose in our body. If blood glucose levels drop too low, for example in patients with type 1 diabetes, this can cause them to become confused and hallucinate.

There are two large categories of carbohydrates, based on their structure: simple and complex.

Simple carbohydrates include sugars like glucose, fructose and sucrose. They are called 'simple' because they contain only one or two units of sugar or saccharides. Their simple make-up means that they are very quickly digested and absorbed into the bloodstream giving us a fast supply of energy. This is why runners and cyclists guzzle down glucose gels and sports drinks during their races for quick energy boosts.

Simple sugars can be found naturally in foods, such as fruit and milk, or as a 'refined' sugar in processed foods, such as sweets, cakes, syrups and fizzy drinks.

Refined sugar from processed foods provides us with a quick energy surge which leaves us bouncing off the walls. While this may sound like a good thing, it doesn't last very long and the aftermath is never very fun. Our body tends to over-correct to bring the level of blood sugar down by releasing a ton of insulin. So suddenly you go from a high level of blood sugar to a low level of blood sugar, which causes feelings of tiredness, irritability and food cravings.

However, simple sugars are not only found in processed foods, but also in many natural foods. For example, fruit contains a simple carbohydrate called fructose, and milk contains a simple carbohydrate called lactose. Sources of natural sugar are considered healthier than refined sugars, because they contain additional nutrients, such as vitamins, minerals and fibre. The fibre content also helps to slow down the absorption of sugar so you don't get such drastic swings in your blood sugar levels. One word of caution: just because it's 'natural' doesn't mean it doesn't contain lots of sugar – or calories. Honey, dates and coconut sugar are all excellent sources of natural sugars but you should still limit your intake – just like you would when adding regular sugar to your tea.

Complex carbohydrates are called polysaccharides, poly meaning many, as they're made up of lots of sugar groups linked together. This complex arrangement means that they take longer to break down, so they provide a stream of energy over a longer period of time. During my dieting days, I believed that cutting out carbohydrates was the key to weight loss. I ditched bread, potatoes, pasta and rice. However, my not understanding carbohydrates meant I was essentially excluding complex carbohydrates from my diet, but still eating simple sugars from foods like sweetened yogurts, cereal bars and dried fruit. I didn't replace the missing carbohydrates with protein or healthy fats so my diet was just sugar and not much else. I felt sluggish, I was always hungry, and I didn't lose weight.

Now I love my carbs, and I know how to choose the right type of carbs that fuel my body and give me energy, but don't send me on a sugar rollercoaster of highs and lows. Most of my carbohydrate intake is now in the form of complex carbohydrates, such as grains, vegetables and legumes. These carbohydrates are also very nutrient dense as they contain important vitamins and minerals, as well as fibre, some protein and also healthy fats.

HOW ARE CARBOHYDRATES USED?

Carbohydrates are first broken down into their simplest form – glucose – and pass into the gut, where they are absorbed into the bloodstream via microvilli, which are like the bristles on a brush, lining the gastrointestinal tract. The presence of sugar in the bloodstream causes the hormone insulin to be released from the pancreas, a gland that sits under your stomach. Insulin acts as a gatekeeper, allowing cells to take up glucose and use it as energy. If not enough insulin is produced, such as in patients with diabetes, the cells cannot get the energy they need from glucose leading to lack of energy and fatigue.

Any excess glucose that is not used as energy is stored as glycogen. This is a type of carbohydrate inside your liver and muscles which we can use as a back-up source of energy. We call on this glucose store if our blood sugar levels are low, for instance, if we haven't eaten in several hours or we have just done a hard workout and used up all our available glucose. When this happens, our trusty pancreas fires back into action but this time releases a hormone called glucagon. This hormone essentially acts in the opposite fashion of insulin and increases circulating blood sugar levels by changing the stored glycogen back into glucose. So that we can now use it as fuel again.

While too much sugar can play havoc with our blood glucose levels, not enough sugar can also have some pretty horrible symptoms. You probably know what I'm talking about if you've gone for a long time without food or worked hard in the gym without breakfast. You may have felt a bit unsteady on your feet, anxious, dizzy, weak, shaky or sweaty. This is why it is important that we include good-quality complex carbohydrates in our diet, particularly when we are active, so that we have enough back-up fuel for when we need it.

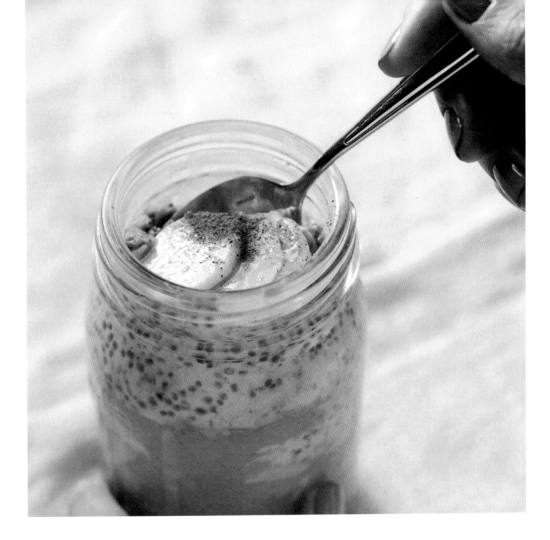

THE BITTER SIDE OF SUGAR

Unfortunately, our modern lifestyles mean we sit more at our desks, in our cars, or in front of the TV. We are moving less, but eating more. If we are sitting down all day and not doing any form of activity, we need less carbohydrates because we are not using up these muscle glycogen stores and therefore don't need to worry about restocking them with a high carbohydrate intake.

Excessive consumption of refined sugar over long periods of time can cause the cells in our body to become resistant to insulin, which results in type 2 diabetes. The cells essentially change their locks so that insulin does not work and glucose cannot enter. The glucose gets stuck in the blood stream and levels begin to rise. More and more insulin is released to try to bring down the high levels of sugar in the blood but eventually the pancreas isn't able to keep up and can't make enough insulin to keep your blood glucose levels normal. This means the cells aren't getting the energy they need and also, over time, high levels of blood glucose cause damage to nerves and blood vessels, leading to complications, such as heart disease, strokes, kidney disease and blindness.

HOW TO BE CARB CLEVER

To help simplify a very complex topic, it may help to think of carbohydrates in terms of a traffic light system:

RED represents refined sugars which are unnatural or processed simple carbohydrates. We should look to limit or remove them from our diet.

AMBER represents simple carbohydrates from nature which are full of beneficial vitamins and minerals, but as they are still sugar, we should monitor our intake.

GREEN represents complex carbohydrates which should make up the bulk of your carbohydrate intake – think fresh greens, wholegrains and legumes.

SIMPLE CARBOHYDRATES (Refined or processed)	SIMPLE CARBOHYDRATES (Natural)	COMPLEX CARBOHYDRATES (Refined or processed)
Chocolate	Fruit	Green vegetables (e.g. *spinach and kale*)
Sweets and cakes	Fruit juice	Wholegrains (e.g. *oats, rye, quinoa, rice*)
Fizzy drinks	Dried fruit	
Sauces and condiments	Honey	Starchy vegetables (e.g. *sweet potato*)
Table sugar	Maple syrup	
Corn syrup and high-frustose corn syrup	Milk and dairy	Beans, lentils and peas
Refined grains (e.g. *white bread*)		
Fruit juice concentrate		

One little clause to add:

We all know that fruit is healthy, so fruit juice must be healthy too? Unfortunately, it really is not that simple. Fruit juice is a key example of how hidden sugars and added calories can sneak into your diet. Per serving, fruit juice requires more fruit, and therefore more sugar, than you would normally consume if you were to eat a piece of fruit. For example, you wouldn't eat ten whole oranges but you could easily drink the juice of ten. On top of the sugar content, many companies include preservatives and flavourings to prolong the shelf-life and improve the flavour of their juices. I'm not telling you to completely cut fruit juices from your diet, but to be wary when choosing a fruit juice from the supermarket. If I fancy a fruit juice, I make my own at home and add in some vegetables to decrease the total sugar content and also to increase the nutritional content.

FIBRE

Non-starch polysaccharides (NSP), better known as fibre, are a little bit different. Dietary fibre is a non-digestible form of carbohydrate so it passes through our digestive system without being absorbed and used as fuel.

SO WHAT IS IT USED FOR THEN?

OK, so complex carbohydrates are about to get even more complex. There are two types of fibre, soluble and insoluble:

SOLUBLE – this includes naturally gel-forming fibres, such as pectins and gums, and is mainly found in the inside of plants. It works by absorbing water in the gut which softens stools making them easier to pass. Grains, such as oats, bran and barley, legumes, such as beans, peas and lentils, and fruit and vegetables like pears, berries, cucumbers and courgettes are rich in soluble fibre.

INSOLUBLE – this fibre is found in the outer layer of plants. It is undigested in the gut, and works by adding bulk to the stool, which improves motility through the gut. It can be found in wholegrains like oats and barley, nuts and seeds, the skin of fruit and vegetables, and popcorn.

SO APART FROM WHAT THEY DO FOR YOUR POO, WHAT ELSE DO THEY DO?

- Lowers blood cholesterol – a large study looking at the results from multiple clinical trials found that diets high in soluble fibre decrease the amount of LDL cholesterol (aka the bad cholesterol) and also decrease the total amount of cholesterol.

- Reduces the risk of cardiovascular disease (CVD) and coronary heart disease (CHD) – fibre can actually reduce the risk of heart disease by improving levels of cholesterol and improving insulin sensitivity.

- Super satiating – eating food high in fibre helps you feel fuller for longer, which helps with maintenance, and even loss, of weight. Adding fibrous vegetables to your meal will not only fill you up, but they tend to be nutrient-dense and low in calories so you really do get more bang for your buck.

- Helps control blood sugar levels – soluble fibre helps to slow down the absorption of glucose and can reduce the initial spike, and subsequent drop, in blood glucose levels so you aren't left feeling lethargic, hungry and craving more sugar.

- **Healthy gut** – although we can't digest and absorb dietary fibre, the bacteria in our gut ferments it and uses it as fuel. We want to keep our gut bacteria happy because these little guys help us to digest food that we can't break down, produce certain nutrients, such as vitamin K, and form a protective barrier against other harmful bugs. Dietary fibre also keeps things moving nice and smoothly through the gut, which reduces the risk of developing haemorrhoids and small pouches in your colon, known as diverticular disease.

HOW MUCH FIBRE SHOULD I BE HAVING?

The Scientific Advisory Committee on Nutrition (SACN) recommend that adults should consume 30g of fibre per day, but currently in the UK we are averaging an intake of about 18g. These numbers are a little redundant if we don't put them into context, so let's take a bowl of porridge as an example:

50G OATS = 4.5G
½ BANANA = 1.5G
HANDFUL OF RASPBERRIES = 4G
TOTAL = APPROXIMATELY 10G OF FIBRE

As we can see, a healthy, balanced diet can provide enough fibre in a day. No one is expecting you to count the grams of fibre in every morsel of food that passes your lips, but it's something to be mindful of, especially if you're feeling a little 'backed-up'.

TIPS FOR INCREASING YOUR FIBRE INTAKE

1 Sneak more veggies into your diet – I LOVE my vegetables, but that wasn't always the case. To help me fall in love with my veggies, I started trying weird and wonderful ways to slip more vegetables into what I was eating. I often add grated courgette to my oats (don't knock it till you've tried it!), kale to my smoothies, and sweet potato to my cakes. This not only adds another source of fibre to the meal, but it also adds an abundance of additional nutrients and volume to the meal, leaving you satisfied for longer.

2 Choose REAL food – are you tired of me repeating this? I honestly cannot reiterate the improvements you can make to your health by choosing unrefined whole foods instead of packaged, processed foods. I always used to peel my fruit and vegetables, and now there's not many that I won't eat the skin of: apples, carrots, butternut squash, potatoes, courgettes and even kiwis.

3 Opt for wholegrain over its white counterpart – wholegrains contain all the essential parts of the grain: the outer bran layer, the inner germ layer and the starchy core. During processing, the bran and the germ are removed to give a 'whiter' cereal. As a result the fibre content is reduced and so is the nutrient content. Wholegrains include:

oats, buckwheat, quinoa, spelt, wheat, rye and barley.

4 Load up on legumes – beans, peas and lentils are among the best sources of fibre out there. Sneak them into your diet by adding them to salads, curries and stews. If you don't have time to soak and cook them, pick up the microwave packets in the supermarket. Wait, she's recommending packaged foods? I know, I know, but in some cases pre-prepared or pre-cooked foods can be really handy when you're trying to juggle a healthy lifestyle with a hectic life. After a long day I often pick up a pack of puy lentils, pop a salmon fillet in the oven, and serve them with some steamed green beans. Remember, eating healthily does not need to be fussy or expensive.

EVER HEARD OF 'TOO MUCH OF A GOOD THING'?

THE SAME APPLIES TO FIBRE.

If you are used to eating a low-fibre diet, increasing your fibre intake may cause you to experience gas and bloating as your gut flora changes and adapts.

When I introduced more fibrous foods like fruit and vegetables to my diet, my digestive system took a couple of weeks to adjust and I had some stomach cramps (and a lot of gas). Keep in mind this was a girl whose only previous source of vegetables was those blended up inside of a tin of soup.

We all react to fibre differently, so if you do feel very uncomfortable, it may be wise to reduce your intake for a couple of days to allow the symptoms to resolve. To prevent this from happening in the first place, slowly increase your fibre intake step-by-step.

Try adding in 2 to 3g per day, about the amount in an unpeeled apple. If you can comfortably tolerate this amount, slowly increase it week by week. On top of this make sure you're drinking enough water and keeping active with regular exercise.

FATS

FATS, GLORIOUS FATS

Thankfully the days of the low-fat fad have ended – for the most part. For so long it was ingrained in society to steer clear of any 'fatty' foods, particularly foods high in saturated fat. Thankfully research has shown that fat is not the enemy. However, I still often hear people adopting a low-fat diet because they believe it is healthier or that it will lead to greater weight loss. It's times like this that I realise we still have a long way to go in the war against the low-fat fanatics.

Walk into any supermarket and 'diet' or 'low-fat' products line the shelves. It's all good and well cutting down on calories, but we're replacing actual foods with processed alternatives with all the best nutrients sucked out of them. I was one of those people who would buy anything labelled 'low-fat', because I was misinformed. I thought I was making the right choices for my health because that's what I read online and in magazines. Now that I know the actual facts, I want to help dispel the myths surrounding dietary fat.

Fat's poor reputation is not only based on the fact that it offers higher energy content per gram in comparison to other macronutrients (i.e. per serving it's more calorific), but primarily because of health concerns surrounding heart disease and cholesterol. Ladies and gentlemen, I'm going to put your mind at rest and debunk the myths using sound scientific evidence. But first, let's talk a little bit about what fat actually is, what it does and where to find it.

WHY IS FAT SO IMPORTANT?

Energy – fat acts as a source of energy for our body, and it can also be stored for times when energy reserves are low and we need fuel.

ABSORPTION OF NUTRIENTS – certain vitamins (A, D, E, K) are fat soluble and are insoluble in blood. Bile acids produced from cholesterol in the liver help to make it bioavailable so the body can absorb it.

HEALTHY NERVES – fats form part of the myelin sheath which is a fatty material that wraps around our nerve cells so that they can send electrical messages between different nerve cells in our body.

BRAIN POWER – essential fatty acids – omega 3 and omega 6 – support brain performance and memory, and also influence behaviour and mood.

SUPPLE SKIN AND SHINY HAIR – maybe she's born with it? Maybe it's omega 3! Supplementing your diet with good-quality fats is the key to glowing skin and glossy hair.

WHAT IS FAT MADE UP OF?

The avocado has essentially become the unofficial logo of health-conscious foodies across the world. From smashed avocado on toast to avocado smoothie bowls, this superfood is the most popular kid on the block right now. We all know it's good for us and many people know it is full of healthy fats, but how many of us know what a healthy fat actually is? Let's take a closer look at the types of fat in our diet.

There are three main types of dietary fat that we need to be aware of: saturated fats, unsaturated fats (monounsaturated and polyunsaturated), and trans fats.

Without boring you too much with the science, what makes a saturated fat different to an unsaturated fat is basically its structure. The simplest unit of fat is the fatty acid. A fatty acid with a single bond is a saturated fat and a fatty acid with a double bond is an unsaturated fat. The structure of these fats is what makes them behave differently in the body and ultimately determines how they impact our health.

• Unsaturated

Unsaturated fats tend to be liquid at room temperature – think olive oils, nut oils, fish oils, but also nuts and seeds.

There are two types of unsaturated fats: monounsaturated (single double bond) and polyunsaturated fatty acids (two or more double bonds).

Monounsaturated

Monounsaturated fats are found in olive and nut oils, avocados, nuts and seeds. Ever wonder why doctors love recommending the monounsaturated-rich Mediterranean diet? Well, a diet high in monounsaturated fats can reduce the amount of LDL (bad) cholesterol, and overall reduce your risk of heart disease, atherosclerosis (plaque in the arteries), high blood pressure and stroke. Swapping monounsaturated fats for refined carbohydrates in your diet can also increase your HDL (or good) cholesterol.

Polyunsaturated

Polyunsaturated fats (PUFAs) are rich in foods, such as oily fish, walnuts, flaxseeds and vegetable oils. The two main PUFAs in our diet are omega 3 and omega 6. These are essential to our diet, so just like the essential amino acids in protein, we need to get them from our food as our bodies cannot make them.

Omega 3 and omega 6 fats are both really important in our diet; however, in recent years, the Western diet has been far more skewed to omega 6 than omega 3 fatty acids. Why is this important? In general, omega 6 fatty acids are pro-inflammatory while omega 3 fatty acids are anti-inflammatory, so a higher ratio of omega 6 to omega 3 means that inflammatory processes in the body are increased. Inflammation is not always a bad thing, it's actually really important for protecting our bodies from infection and injury, but as with anything in excess, it can be harmful. It's believed that this excess consumption of omega 6 is one of the leading drivers behind today's increase in inflammatory diseases, such as cardiovascular disease, inflammatory bowel disease, rheumatoid arthritis, and Alzheimer's disease.

What I want you to take away from this is that a diet that is high in omega 6 but low in omega 3 increases inflammation, so focus on increasing your omega 3 intake to help balance it out. I've included all the best sources of omega 3 in the table on page 37.

- **Saturated fats**

Saturated fats tend to be solid at room temperature – think butter, coconut oil and steak. I'm sure you've heard of saturated fat, and for all the wrong reasons too.

When I was at school we were taught that fats were either: good fats (monounsaturated), very good fats (polyunsaturated) or bad fats (saturated and trans fats). This has largely been the worldwide consensus since the 1950s when an American scientist, Ancel Keys, published a study where he found association between dietary saturated fat intake and increased risk of heart disease. This was only an association, which means he found a relationship between saturated fat and heart disease, but there could be other things affecting the relationship that he didn't take into consideration – such as carbohydrate intake. So the evidence wasn't very convincing to start off with. Keys also excluded some of the data which didn't fit with his findings to make his results look better. Despite scientists picking holes in his flawed research, public health authorities across the world integrated his advice into their guidelines and encouraged people to reduce their saturated fat intake.

This low-fat hype has led to increased consumption of processed foods in which fat has been replaced by sugar, sweeteners and other chemicals, in order to make up for the

---

SO WHAT ARE THE FACTS?

Well, saturated fat does raise the bad LDL cholesterol, but it also raises the good HDL cholesterol. So this means that our total cholesterol (i.e. HDL + LDL) is high. However, total cholesterol gives you no indication of how much is good and how much is bad. You can have high total cholesterol, but if a large percentage of it is made of up of HDL, then your risk of cardiovascular disease is low. Overall the cholesterol ratio (total cholesterol/HDL cholesterol) improves, which is a more useful marker of heart disease risk.

Before you start reaching for the cheese board, this does not mean that a high saturated fat intake is completely harmless. When I indulge in saturated fats, it's usually in the form of some good-quality fillet steak or good-quality 85 per cent dark chocolate. I don't eat very much of it and I may not eat it every day but it's certainly something that I don't exclude from my diet. Like all types of fat, it has a high calorie content and eating too much of it will cause you to gain weight.

- **Trans fats**

If there is any fat that we should be avoiding, it's this bad boy. Trans fats are created by artificially hardening unsaturated fats through a process called 'hydrogenation'. Companies do this to improve the texture and prolong the shelf life – good for business, but not for health. Trans fats increase levels of bad cholesterol, reduce levels of good cholesterol, promote weight gain, and increase our risk of heart disease. So how do you avoid them? Cut out processed foods like biscuits, sweets, margarines, pies and pastries, and fried food, which are soaked in the stuff.

SO HOW MUCH FAT SHOULD WE BE HAVING?

In the UK, the guidelines state that no more than 35 per cent of total daily calories should come from fat and only 11 per cent of this should come from saturated fat. As we now know, saturated fat is not as bad for us as we once thought, and it can actually be beneficial to our health – in the right amounts. So again, when it comes to saturated fat intake, the age-old phrase of 'everything in moderation' definitely holds true. But please, keep it simple. Don't worry too much about exact percentages and grams. What I want you to do is:

- Avoid industrially processed and artificially created trans fats.

- Get most of your dietary fat from sources which are rich in monounsaturated and polyunsaturated fats, such as avocados, olive oil, nuts and seeds, and oily fish.

- Load up on omega 3 rich foods such as salmon, flaxseed and walnuts.

- When eating saturated fat, choose good-quality foods, such as extra-virgin coconut oil, grass-fed beef and full-fat, unsweetened Greek yogurt.

TRANS FATS	SATURATED	MONO-UNSATURATED	POLYUNSATURATED	
			Omega 6	Omega 3
Cakes and biscuits Margarines Takeaways Pies and pastries Fried food	Meat Full-fat dairy Coconut Coconut oil Palm oil	Olive oil Avocados Peanut oil Rapeseed oil Nuts and seeds	Sunflower oil Soya bean oil Rapeseed oil	Oily fish Flaxseed Walnuts

NUTRITION MYTHS

I want to bust some of the myths out there about health – the info here should help sort the facts from the fads.

1. GLUTEN IS HARMFUL AND FATTENING

Gluten is the dietary villain of this decade, just like carbohydrates were to the 90s and fat was to the 70s. Take a look at the menu of any 'healthy' cafe nowadays and you will struggle to find a cake or dessert that contains gluten. Many people can justify eating a cake that contains refined sugar, just because it's gluten-free . . . so it must be healthy, right?

Increased awareness and media coverage of gluten, the good and the bad, has led to an increased availability of gluten-free products on the market. This is great news for those who have to avoid gluten for medical reasons because the availability of gluten-free alternatives makes social events much less isolating. However, it seems to have caused a wave of panic across the nation and many of us are voluntarily going gluten-free after self-diagnosing online because it's perceived to be healthier, or because it's simply 'trendy' right now.

To set the record straight: for the majority of us, gluten isn't harmful. Gluten is essentially a family of proteins found in certain grains, such as wheat, rye and barely. It gives dough that glue-like consistency which makes for perfect soft, chewy breads, bagels and pizzas. It's perfectly natural, but for people with coeliac disease, gluten sensitivity or the much less common skin condition, dermatitis herpetiformis, it can be harmful.

People with coeliac disease have a serious reaction to gluten where their body's defence system mistakes the gluten as a threat and produces antibodies to fight it. This reaction damages the surface of the small bowel, interfering with the body's ability to absorb nutrients from food. Coeliac disease is an autoimmune disease, not a food allergy or a food intolerance. In an autoimmune disease, the immune system (the body's defence system) mistakes something harmless, like gluten, to be harmful. Coeliac disease affects 1 in 100 people in the UK and Europe. It is diagnosed by a special blood test which checks for the antibodies to gluten, or by a biopsy of the small bowel. The only cure for the disease is a lifelong gluten-free diet.

People with coeliac disease tend to get very sick, very quickly if they eat even the most microscopic amount of gluten. Other people may have 'intolerances' or 'sensitivity' to gluten where they suffer from some discomfort after eating gluten, such as diarrhoea and bloating, but do not actually have coeliac disease. For a long time, the medical view of gluten intolerance was black or white: either you have coeliac disease or you don't. However, gluten sensitivity, or non coeliac gluten sensitivity (NCGS), is becoming increasingly recognised by the healthcare profession as a separate diagnosis. NCGS is a diagnosis of exclusion, whereby people experience symptoms after eating foods containing gluten but the tests for coeliac disease are negative. The issue is that there is no formal test to diagnose NCGS so many healthcare practitioners are still on the fence as to whether it actually exists. Personally

All of my recipes give gluten-free options so that you can substitute ingredients depending on your requirements.

I believe it's hardly an all-or-nothing affair, and from reading the research and speaking to patients, it's clear that some people really do experience physical symptoms from consuming gluten. The wishy-washy diagnosis means that it often goes unrecognised, but nowadays my feeling is that it's maybe over-diagnosed due to the amount of people self-diagnosing. I think part of the reason for this is because of how gluten is portrayed in the media as a toxic substance which apparently pokes holes in the lining of your gut.

If you don't have coeliac disease and you don't have issues with gluten, then removing gluten from your diet will have no effect on your health. I promise you that it's not fattening in any shape or form, and it's not going to kill you. The idea that a 'gluten-free' label equates to healthy or nutritious is not true. Gluten-free products can be just as heavily processed as any other type of food. A brownie is still a brownie, gluten-free or not. They both have refined sugar, trans fats, additives, preservatives and flavourings – and calories. We need to focus less on cutting out foods from our diet and focus more on what we need to be including in our diets – real food.

2. PROTEIN SHAKES WILL MAKE ME BULKY

From all the people who have come to me for advice, particularly women, there seems to be this common misconception that having a protein shake will cause superhuman muscle gains.

For anyone who may be avoiding protein supplements for the fear that they may gain weight or 'bulk' up, I would like to reassure you now that that's really not the case. First of all, gaining muscle is a lot harder than it may seem – it requires weight training, a high calorie diet and consistency.

Secondly, having a protein shake is just like having any other source of lean protein. Let's compare it to a chicken breast: they both contain roughly the same amount of protein, both are low in fat, and the calories in each are not too dissimilar. The biggest advantage of a protein shake is the convenience, and also how cost-effective they are.

Although protein shakes were initially marketed for people to drink straight after they work out, that's not the only time when they come in handy. If you don't have time for breakfast in the morning, then whipping up a smoothie with a scoop of protein is a quick way to ensure you're getting some protein into you before heading off to work. They're also a great addition or substitute when baking healthy cakes and snacks. With that said, I'm a firm believer in food first, but if you're struggling to meet your daily protein targets through diet alone then protein supplements are a great, convenient way to fill in the gaps. First and foremost, base your meals around good-quality sources of protein, such as lean meat and poultry, egg whites, fish and dairy.

3. EATING FAT MAKES YOU FAT AND ILL

The media, food industry and healthcare systems across the world have named and shamed saturated fat consumption as one of the biggest risk factors for the development of obesity and associated cardiovascular disease.

However, despite the strict protocol of a low-fat diet – as outlined by national dietary advice – levels of cardiovascular disease, cholesterol and the nation's waistband has continued to increase. But is fat really to blame?

I think we've made leaps and bounds in terms of changing our opinion on dietary fat and health, but it seems like this little misconception tends to still pop up now and then – even in government guidelines. The bottom line is: fat doesn't make you fat, excess calories make you fat. The fat that you eat in food does not automatically get transported to the tissue on your body, any more than eating more protein will automatically build muscle.

It's a different kettle of fish if we are referring to the trans fats we find in junk food. These fats are certainly not good for your health or your waistline. So don't fear fat, but choose good-quality sources, such as eggs, avocados, nuts and seeds, oily fish, extra-virgin olive oil, coconut oil and grass-fed meat. Repeat after me: fat is friend, not foe.

4. FRUCTOSE IS BAD FOR YOU

First it was fat, now it's fructose – we are constantly searching for a macronutrient to blame for the surge in obesity and diabetes. However, time and time again, the only solid conclusion we can come to is that any food group in excess can lead to weight gain.

You've probably heard of fructose as the sugar that comes from fruit; however, most of our daily fructose nowadays comes from non-fruit sources, usually in the form of a sweetener known as high fructose corn syrup (HFCS). This sweetener is found in processed foods, such as sweets, fizzy drinks and sugary cereals. The consumption of HFCS has increased over the past few decades, which coincides with the increase in obesity, diabetes and cardiovascular disease. The conclusion has largely been that fructose consumption, as part of a normal diet, doesn't have much of an impact on our health but when fructose is eaten in excess (i.e. on top of a normal diet), this increases our calorie intake, which in turn leads to weight gain and other health problems like obesity and diabetes. In short, anything in excess isn't good for you and will cause you to put on weight.

There is nothing uniquely bad or fattening about fructose compared to any other nutrient. If eaten as part of a normal healthy diet. Sugary drinks cause weight gain and health issues because it's easy to over-consume on calories and not realise it. So my biggest piece of advice would be to avoid sugary drinks and concentrated fruit juices, and focus on getting good-quality carbohydrates through fruit and vegetables.

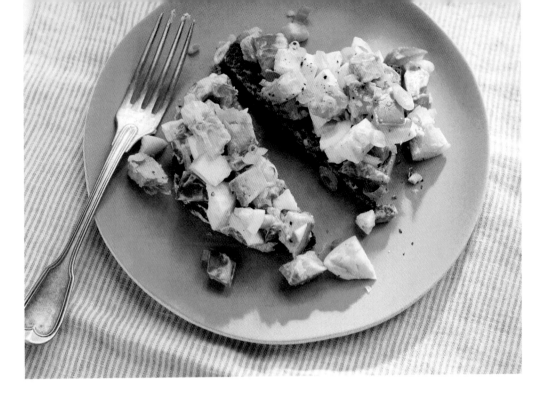

5. EAT SIX SMALL MEALS A DAY TO BOOST YOUR METABOLISM

Sound familiar? I've certainly heard and read this in the media hundreds of times. I also tried it out myself a couple of years ago, and instead of losing weight I actually put on weight because I just ended up eating the same size meals – but more of them.

The theory is that eating more meals a day increases your metabolism, and therefore burns more calories. When we eat food, and digest it, we actually do use energy, and therefore burn calories. This is called the thermic effect of food (TEF), and equals about 10 per cent of total calorie intake. However, this varies from person to person, and the total amount of calories consumed, not how many meals you eat, is the most important factor when we are looking to lose weight. Eating six 250-calorie meals a day, as opposed to three 500-calorie meals, still equates to 1,500-calories at the end of the day.

Eating six smaller meals may benefit you if you struggle with hunger and cravings throughout the day, but keep in mind that if you're increasing the number of meals you need to decrease the size of the meals so that you're not eating an excessive amount of calories.

In terms of convenience, it can also be pretty tricky to fit six meals into a working day. With my hectic days on the ward, I cannot always guarantee that I will get a break when I planned to so I personally prefer to have my three standard meals – breakfast, lunch and dinner – and then have two snacks as and when I can fit them in.

Fundamentally, meal frequency really isn't something to be too concerned about – it's more the amount of calories you consume. You can eat several smaller meals across the day, or you can space them out and eat fewer, larger meals. The best healthy diet is the one that you're going to stick to so decide what works best for you and your lifestyle.

6. 'CLEAN' FOODS VS 'DIRTY' FOODS

The words we use to describe food are more important than many of us realise. It not only affects what we eat but how we feel after we eat it.

Attaching words like 'clean' or 'guilt-free' to certain foods, and 'dirty' or 'cheat' to others implies that certain foods are off limits and those who eat those foods are unclean and should feel guilty. Like many others, I've used 'clean-eating' synonymously with 'healthy-eating' without really thinking through the consequences. Typically, clean foods are considered to be natural and unprocessed foods, like fruit and vegetables, and dirty foods tend to be high-calorie, processed foods, like pizza and chocolate. Other people may use the phrase 'clean-eating' to represent their own dietary choices, i.e. vegan or paleo (see Glossary). So one person's idea of what foods are 'clean' doesn't necessarily reflect another person's idea – this leads to judgement and fear about what we should or shouldn't be consuming, which, for some people, can lead to unhealthy and obsessive behaviour around food.

At the time of this book going to print, there were more than 27,000,000 Instagram posts with the hashtag #cleaneating. The success of this movement is largely to do with the exponential surge in the number of health and fitness accounts. All those colourful, mouthwatering photos of green juices, smashed avo on toast and raw desserts are enough to convince anyone to jump on the bandwagon and invest in a spiraliser. While there's nothing wrong with a little healthy eating inspiration, I worry about the language used and the 'tips' given by people who are not qualified to give such advice.

Yes, there are certain foods that are, from a nutritional stand point, a better option – for example, an apple vs a slice of cake. However, if you fancy a slice of birthday cake that does not make you a bad person and you should enjoy it without having the need to label it a 'cheat' or a 'guilty pleasure'.

I also fear that those who try to adhere strictly to their 'clean-eating' rules will end up restricting important food groups, missing out on nutrients, negatively impacting their social life, and ultimately developing an unhealthy relationship with food – the opposite of what they probably intended to achieve in the first place.

My philosophy is everything in moderation. I love eating whole foods like fresh fruit and vegetables, because I know that they make me feel good, fill me with energy and nourish my body with all their vitamins and minerals. On the flip side, I also love salty chip shop chips, cheesy nachos, and tubs of ice cream. I don't consider them off-limits or 'dirty' but I'm certainly not tucking into them every day because I know that although they may taste good and make me happy, they don't fill me with energy and they lack many essential nutrients. Food is much more than a source of energy – it's a part of our heritage, it's tradition, it brings friends and family together.

7. DON'T EAT CARBS AFTER SIX

This is probably one of the oldest 'tips' in the book.

The reasoning behind this theory is that eating carbs late at night will cause them to store as fat due to your metabolism slowing down as you go to sleep. On the other hand, if they are eaten during the day when you are busy and active, they get burned off. While it's true your metabolism slows down when you go to sleep, it doesn't stop, and your body is still functioning behind the scenes while you're asleep.

If you exclude starchy carbohydrates from your dinner, such as rice, potato or pasta, and don't replace it with other food groups, you're ultimately reducing the amount of calories in the meal. So the secret isn't cutting carbs; the reason people may lose weight following this rule is simply because they're reducing their total calorie intake.

As we know, carbohydrates have an important role in our diet and act as the body's main source of fuel. Certain carbohydrates, particularly complex carbs, are also very nutrient-dense and packed full of fibre. This not only provides you with important vitamins and minerals, but it also fills you up so you're less likely to snack in the night.

8. YOU CAN DETOX YOUR BODY THROUGH CLEANSES, TEAS OR JUICE DIETS

The term 'detox' means detoxification, which is a normal process carried out by the body to remove toxic substances, such as waste products like ammonia, medication and other drugs, and alcohol. This word is often misused as a buzzword for 'cleansing' or 'flushing out' toxins from our body with the use of supplements or foods.

Detox diets range from juice cleanses and 'skinny' teas to colon cleanses and enemas. They claim to remove harmful toxins that build up in your body – these toxins are said to cause nasty side effects like weight gain, health problems and even cancer. However, none of these claims are scientifically backed up and it's a wonder these products even made it to the shelves.

What makes matters even worse is that many of these 'cleanses' can actually be very dangerous. Many detox teas and other weight loss supplements contain laxatives, which stimulate a bowel movement, and diuretics, which promote the production of urine. They can cause dehydration, and depletion of important minerals, such as sodium, potassium and calcium.

My advice? Steer clear of anything that claims to 'detox' or 'cleanse'. We have an in-built detox system in our body. The foods that we eat, the air that we breathe and the things that we touch mean that we come into contact with toxins like chemicals and pollutants every day. Our body, mainly the liver, filters these toxins and passes them out of our bodies through our sweat, urine and faeces. Having a green juice or slapping on a detox patch to your foot isn't going to speed up the process.

CALORIES

A calorie is the unit we use to measure the amount of energy that we get from food.

CALORIES = ENERGY

Have you ever seen one of those advertisements with a chocolate bar and the number of minutes on the treadmill you have to do in order to burn it off? First of all, exercise should not be a punishment for something you ate, and second, we don't just burn calories when we exercise. You are burning calories just reading the words on this page and turning the pages of this book. Let me explain . . .

AT REST

The body requires energy (i.e. calories) just to function. Calories are used to pump blood around the body, to breathe, to keep us warm, to digest our food, to blink, to talk, to think! The amount of energy (or calories) that we need for our bodies to function at rest is known as the basal metabolic rate, or BMR. This is why people who severely undereat become very sick – their bodies struggle to carry out normal everyday functions and we see signs like dizziness, cold intolerance, dry skin, loss of hair and the cessation of menstrual periods in women.

EATING FOOD

Eating also requires calories to chew, swallow, digest, absorb and uses the food for fuel. But before you get too excited – it's only about 5–15 per cent of your calorie intake and it differs for each food group. The food groups that burn the most calories are protein and fibre, because they take longer to break down and be used by the body. This is believed to be the reason high protein diets cause greater weight loss compared to diets equal in calories but higher in carbohydrates.

DURING EXERCISE

Finally, as we already know, we burn calories when we exercise!

So bringing this all together, the total energy you use in a day is the sum of the calories you burn at rest, from food, and from exercise. In order to lose weight we need to make sure that we are burning more calories than we are eating. Vice versa, if we eat more food than we need and don't use those extra calories, we gain weight!

IS A CALORIE JUST A CALORIE?

Regardless of which foods the calories come from, if we eat roughly 500 fewer calories per day or burn 500 extra calories per day through exercise, or some combination of the two, we will lose about 1lb a week.

LET'S PUT THIS INTO PERSPECTIVE:

Person A and person B both want to lose weight and both eat 2,500kcal every day. The only difference is person A eats a diet solely of chocolate, and person B eats a balanced diet of protein, carbs and fats. In theory, if they both reduced their daily calorie intake to 2,000kcal, they would lose weight.

I know what you're thinking: so why can't we just go on a diet that consists of chocolate?

Well, both diets may offer us the same amount of fuel but they differ hugely in the quality of fuel. Certain foods fill us up more than others without being full of calories (i.e. fruit, vegetables and lean protein), while other foods are packed full of calories and fail to fill us up (i.e. sweets, cakes and fizzy drinks). This is why it's so easy to overeat on a diet full of junk food! Processed foods are designed to make you want more – they're addictive. I mean, have you ever stopped at just one or two crisps or managed just a nibble of a chocolate bar before putting it away? If so, then you're superhuman, my friend.

Remember, the best diet is the one you can stick to but also one that makes you look and feel great, and something that keeps you out of hospital! Processed foods lack the vitamins and minerals that we need for our bodies to function, not to mention to maximise health!

I want you to switch your focus from the quantity of calories, and instead focus on the quality of calories. Focus on eating a diet full of lean protein, wholesome carbohydrates and healthy fats – the type of food that is rich in vitamins and minerals, makes you strong, gets you lean, gives you energy, and keeps you healthy.

Instead of counting calories, I'm going to show you my easy step-by-step guide to building a balanced plate. This way you will be able to personalise and have fun with the meals that you create, while ensuring that you get a healthy balance of all the food groups. This template is how I build all my meals and create all my recipes. It's really simple, but effective – trust me!

If you don't feel like you're seeing results after a couple of weeks, I want you to put on your detective hat and do some investigating. Keep a food diary for a week and look at your calorie intake to see what your average is. If you want to get really nerdy about it, check how much protein, carbs and fats you're having. If one macronutrient seems to be consistently very high, reduce it. We all respond to certain macronutrients differently, so despite what the science says, it's also very important to listen to your body.

BUILDING A BALANCED PLATE

Now that we have talked through the basics of nutrition, and why each macronutrient is important, you have a good solid foundation of knowledge to start building your own healthy diet. You may not realise it, but you now have the power to make healthy, educated choices about food when you're out shopping, looking through the fridge for dinner choices, and prepping your lunches. I realise it's a lot of information to take on board, so let's pull all of it together and talk through, step-by-step, how to make a balanced meal.

STEP 1 PALM SIZE OF PROTEIN

One way of ensuring that you're meeting your protein goals is by counting your 'macros'. Macros or macronutrients, as explained earlier, include carbohydrates, proteins and fats. For example, one chicken breast has roughly 30g of protein and one egg has roughly 6g of protein. Just as a reminder, we need to be aiming for, at the very least, 0.75g of protein per kg of body weight per day and, for those of us who are physically active and interested in building and maintaining muscle tissue, this should be increased to 1.2–1.7g of protein per kg. So for your average 70kg person, roughly 100g of protein is the perfect target. Personally, I aim for the higher intake of 1.7g per kg, not only for all the benefits listed, but because protein is really satiating so it keeps me fuller for longer and personally, I love protein-rich foods, such as chicken, eggs and whey protein. One thing to point out is that super-exceeding your protein intake will not make your muscles grow any bigger or any faster, so try to aim for your daily requirements but you don't need to go over and above that. How do I know I'm hitting my daily protein goal? I eyeball it using the size of my palm as an approximate measure for each serving of protein.

Personally, I like to base my meals around my protein. If I'm having one serving of protein for my three main meals a day, plus any additional protein in my snacks, then I know I've roughly hit my protein goals for the day. To put it into perspective, let's break it down:

> **BREAKFAST:** 2 eggs, 40g feta cheese **(20g)**
> **LUNCH:** chicken breast **(30g)**
> **DINNER:** salmon fillet **(25g)**
> **SNACK:** small tub of Greek yogurt + handful of nuts **(20g)**
>
> **20 + 30 + 25 + 20 = 95g protein***

This is just an approximation and obviously it excludes other incomplete sources of protein, such as legumes, grains and vegetables.

So for a female of my size and weight, I am consuming roughly 1.8g of protein per kg of body weight which is ideal for my activity levels, and goals to maintain and build muscle mass. For a male who is twice my body weight, then two palm-sized servings of protein would be more suitable in order to ensure that his daily protein macronutrient needs are met. Even for those who live less active lives, I would still recommend maximising your protein intake.

* Estimation only

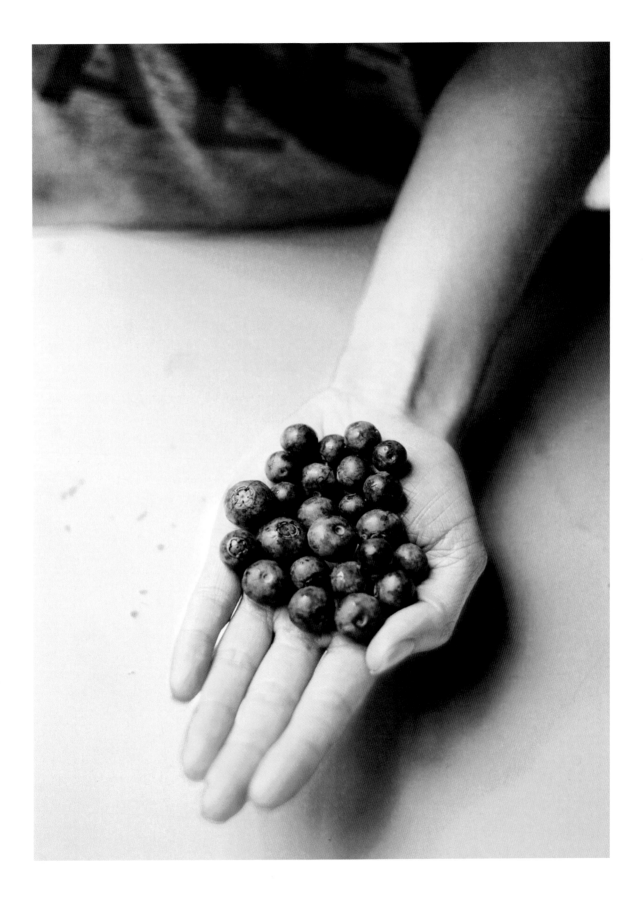

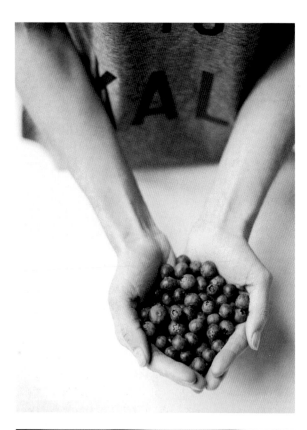

Don't eat anything you can't pronounce . . . except quinoa, you shoud always eat quinoa

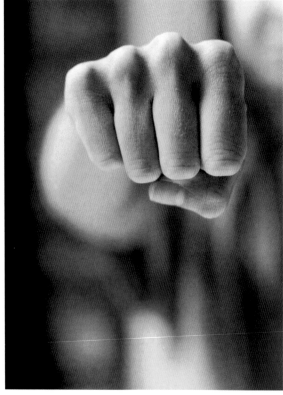

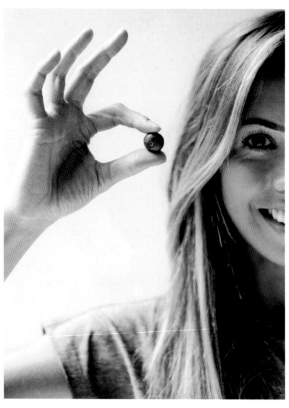

STEP 2 CHOOSE TWO CUPPED HANDS OF NON-STARCHY, FIBROUS VEGETABLES

Non-starchy vegetables, such as leafy greens, broccoli, cauliflower, peppers, cucumbers, carrots, mushrooms and celery, are packed full of nutrients and fibre. They are also lower in calories than starchy vegetables like potatoes and squash, so you can benefit from their goodness by packing out your meals with them, when trying to maintain or lose weight. Add a variety of colour, texture and nutrients to your plate by combining a mixture of vegetables, such as peppers, kale, beetroot and courgette.

When preparing my meals, I always choose at least two or three different types of non-starchy vegetables. The vegetables you choose come down entirely to personal preference but a rule that I like to go by is choosing one leafy green, such as kale, spinach or rocket leaves, and two different coloured vegetables, like aubergine and courgette, for example. You should add two handfuls, or fill half of your plate, with these nutrient-dense foods.

STEP 3 A CLENCHED FIST OF COMPLEX CARBOHYDRATES

Although starchy foods, such as potatoes and rice, are higher in calories and carbohydrates per serving compared to non-starchy vegetables, they are still rich in important vitamins and minerals. Starchy vegetables are also a great source of fibre, and as we know dietary fibre staves off hunger by keeping you feeling fuller for longer. This makes you less likely to have dips in your blood sugar throughout the day so you're less likely to pick and graze on snacks to keep your energy levels up. I think many people still have 'carbophobia' when

it comes to starchy carbs – although hopefully I've helped dispel some of the myths when it comes to them. All carbohydrates are not created equal and choosing the right kind of carbohydrates makes all the difference. Wholesome starchy carbohydrates, which are unrefined and unprocessed, like a whole sweet potato with the skin on or brown rice which hasn't been stripped of its nutritious coat, are nutritionally dense, digested slower and provide us with energy over longer periods of time. The opposite is true of their processed counterparts – foods which are generally white, refined and contain a huge list of weird and wonderful ingredients.

STEP 4 A PINCH OF FAT

A decade ago, low-fat diets were considered the way to go in order to lose weight and prevent heart disease. However, there has been a huge 180 degree turn around in recent years and we now appreciate how essential it is to consume dietary fats for our overall health and well-being. On the whole, this is a very positive thing, but as with everything – too much of a good thing is never a good thing. Unfortunately fat, regardless of how healthy it is, still has calories. It provides over double the calories per gram than that of carbohydrates or protein which means we don't need as much of it in terms of weight, compared to the other macronutrients.

I like to use fats to accessorise my meals – a little drizzle of extra-virgin olive oil, ½ a smashed avocado, a sprinkle of seeds or a dollop of almond butter offers me the nutritional benefits of fat, enhances the flavour of my food, but doesn't add an excessive amount of calories to the meal.

Below is an example of some of the best sources of each macronutrient. The list for fruit and vegetables is endless and in terms of nutrition, you can be as flexible and as creative as you wish when adding these foods to your meal. This comes with a clause: certain fruits are very concentrated forms of sugar, particularly dried fruit, bananas and pineapple. When choosing these fruits, be less generous with your serving. It's easy to munch on a handful of dried apricots but you would never sit and eat ten fresh apricots in one sitting.

PROTEIN	VEGETABLES & FRUIT	COMPLEX CARBOHYDRATES	FATS
Chicken	Spinach	Sweet potato	Nuts
Turkey	Kale	White potato	Seeds
Steak	Pak choi	Butternut squash	Nut butter (1 tsp)
Lean beef mince	Mixed lettuce	Rice	Olive oil (1 tbsp)
Salmon	Broccoli	Quinoa	Grass-fed butter
Tuna	Courgette/courgetti	Oats	Avocado
Eggs	Green beans	Spelt	
Whey/casein	Tomatoes	Barley	
protein	Cucumber	Rye Bread	
Tofu*	Beetroot		
Legumes/beans*	Celery		
Plant-based proteins	Asparagus		
Powders*	Aubergine		
Quark			
Cottage cheese	Berries		
Greek yogurt	Apple		
	Citrus fruits		
	Pear		
	Peach		
	Melon		
	Watermelon		
	Kiwi		
	Banana		

(Include protein (g) per 100 (g))

* Remember, plant-based protein, such as tofu, beans and lentils, are a good source of amino acids, but individually are not 'complete' protein sources. To ensure you're benefiting from all the essential amino acids, combine different beans and pulses together.

SUGAR

Is this the missing macronutrient? I have purposely excluded chocolate, sweets and syrups, such as agave and honey. These foods are non-essential to our diet (maybe essential for the soul) so eat them sparingly but don't consider them as building blocks in your healthy diet.

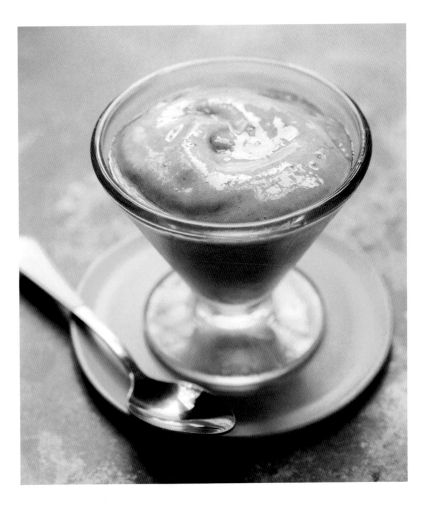

'Let food be thy medicine and medicine be thy food'

HIPPOCRATES

NUTRITION AND DISEASE

The 'father of medicine', Hippocrates practised a holistic approach to medicine.

On the day of graduation, it is tradition for newly qualified doctors to swear by the Hippocratic oath – an ethical and professional declaration, and a promise to, above all, put the patient and their well-being first.

At medical school, we were taught to always act in the best interests of the patient in order to improve their health. We spend years learning how to assess, investigate, diagnose and manage illnesses to improve health and prolong life. Advances in medicine mean that we have a drug or intervention for nearly every condition in the book and if we don't, we're working hard to find one through ongoing research and clinical trials. Levels of mortality have plummeted since the discovery of revolutionary advances, such as immunisations, antibiotics and chemotherapy. As a result we are living longer lives – but not necessarily longer, healthier lives.

Nutrition and our overall health are so intimately linked, yet what we feed our body is often overlooked as the potential culprit to our health problems. It is also often disregarded as a potential solution or prevention to some of our ailments. Food is a double-edged sword – the food we consume acts as fuel for our bodies to help it survive and thrive. If we provide it with good fuel, it will perform at its best, but if we feed it with the wrong type of fuel over a long period of time, the body begins to struggle and so it compensates by making sacrifices elsewhere – sort of like putting diesel in a petrol car. Over time these deficiencies and imbalances can lead to poor health and disease. I'm not just talking about heart disease and obesity, but mental health conditions, such as depression and anxiety, digestive problems, such as malabsorption and diarrhoea, and even skin conditions, such as acne and psoriasis.

In medicine, we are very good at detective work – we diagnose the problem and we try to fix it. The focus has been on finding a cure, treating the symptoms or at least slowing down the progression of disease and illnesses. However, what if we could nip it in the bud before it happens? We all know that prevention is better than cure, so why aren't we practising what we preach? There are some things that influence our health that we can't completely change, like our genetics, but there are things that we do have the control to change – our diet and lifestyle. If we approach the problem from a different angle, we can work forwards to prevent it from happening in the first place, instead of working backwards to find the source of the problem.

THE HEART AND BLOOD VESSELS

The leading cause of death a hundred years ago was infections like influenza and tuberculosis, or 'consumption' as it was once called. Deaths caused by heart disease and associated conditions like diabetes were essentially non-existent. Fast forward a century and now cardiovascular disease causes over 25 per cent of all deaths in the UK – at an average of 425 people each day or one every three minutes.

WHAT IS CARDIOVASCULAR DISEASE?

Cardiovascular disease (CVD) is an umbrella term for all diseases of the heart and blood vessels, including coronary heart disease, stroke and high blood pressure.

CVD happens when fatty deposits and plaque build up on the inside of arteries and cause narrowing, a process called atherosclerosis. The arteries become more and more narrow over time, making it difficult for oxygen-rich blood to pass through. Sometimes a piece of the plaque breaks away from the vessel wall and forms a clot in the artery, completely stopping the blood flow to important organs. If a clot lodges in an artery in the heart, it causes a heart attack, and in the brain, it causes a stroke.

I've been unfortunate to lose my dad to a stroke, and I come across patients every day who have been diagnosed with cardiovascular disease, or at least some of the risk factors. My dad had high blood pressure, and he wasn't very compliant with his medication. He was also pre-diabetic, meaning he had higher blood sugars than normal but not high enough to meet the criteria. The diagnosis of high blood pressure and the potential diagnosis of type 2 diabetes terrified my father. He knew these risk factors were largely lifestyle-related and he was determined to improve his prognosis through diet and exercise. He went to the gym every day and cut back on cakes, sweet treats,

and his nightly routine of wine and cheese. He lost weight, improved his blood cholesterol and was able to manage his blood sugar levels without medication. However, the plaque build-up in his carotid arteries, the arteries in your neck that supply blood to your brain, was too extensive and required more than lifestyle changes alone to fix, but rather surgical intervention.

I don't know if it was too little too late, and I often think about what would have happened if he had changed his lifestyle sooner. I can't dwell on what I could have done to change the fate of my father's outcome, but if I can help prevent another family from losing their father, or their mother, to cardiovascular disease, then I'm certainly going to do my best. My father's death changed my life, it had such an impact on me and it was the biggest driving force behind my decision to become a doctor.

There are many risk factors that cause atherosclerosis, some of which we can't change, like our family history, ethnicity and age. However, other risk factors we do have the power to change. These include: high blood pressure, high cholesterol, obesity, inactivity, type 2 diabetes and smoking. Despite having the power to reduce these risk factors as individuals, we seem to have done nothing about it over the past 100 years – and if anything, we've just made things worse.

SO WHAT HAS CHANGED BETWEEN THEN AND NOW?

Our ancestors had very physical jobs which involved moderate to high levels of activity, meaning they didn't sit for long periods of time and travelled from A to B mainly by foot. Their diets were comprised of basic whole foods sourced from nature, such as meat, fish, nuts, fruit and vegetables. Meals were cooked from scratch with minimal processing, if any at all.

Fast forward to the twenty-first century and the picture looks a little different: most of us work from a desk, we drive cars and catch trains to work, we spend the majority of our spare time sitting down watching TV, or playing on our phones and tablets. Food is always available in the form of ready meals, takeaways and deliveries via apps on our phones. Many of us don't know how to cook from scratch or simply do not have the time to do so – and why bother when we can order our favourite dish with one swipe?

In many ways, the advances we have made in recent years have made the world a safer place to live in – safer from many deadly, once incurable, diseases, safer from accidents and major incidents, and safer from crime and violence. However, in many ways the world is becoming more dangerous due to poor nutrition, inactivity and other lifestyle-related risks, such as smoking and excessive alcohol consumption. With the surge in diseases related to diet and lifestyle, the importance of food cannot be underplayed. If used in the right way, we can help to prevent disease, and even death, with the right dietary and lifestyle changes.

• Omega 3

So you may have gathered by now that I'm a little bit obsessed with healthy fats like omega 3 – but seriously, it does our bodies so much good, especially our hearts. I take Omega 3 daily in the form of cod liver oil supplements. Unfortunately, for years we associated dietary fat with high cholesterol and heart disease. As we now know, these recommendations were based on poor evidence in the 1950s. However, I believe that there are still quite a lot of people, particularly of the older generation, who fear fat because of the perceived health risks and also the misconception that fat makes you fat. Like too much of anything, too much fat will make you fat, but that is because of the excess calories. There is nothing uniquely fattening about fat – despite what many of us have been led to believe.

Omega 3 fatty acids should be a key component in everyone's diet. As it is an essential fatty acid, our bodies can't make it so we need to get it through food. There are actually three different types of omega 3: ALA (alpha-linolenic acid), DHA (docosahexaenoic acid) and EPA (eicosapentaenoic acid). Cardiovascular disease is associated with chronic, or long-term, inflammation in the body. The omega 3 fatty acids, EPA and DHA in particular, support heart health by decreasing inflammation, preventing clot formation, and helping to maintain healthy blood pressure and cholesterol levels.

The recommendations are that we should eat at least two portions of fatty fish, such as salmon and mackerel, a week. All fish and shellfish contain small amounts of mercury, a metal which can be found in nature but is also generated by humans via environmental pollution. This doesn't pose a problem to our health in very small amounts, but as a precaution, pregnant and breastfeeding women should eat no more than two portions of oily fish per week. In addition to fish, omega 3 can be found in foods like walnuts, flaxseed and chia seeds, or supplements like cod liver oil capsules.

• Dietary fibre

If I'm not ranting and raving over how amazing omega 3 is, I'm probably singing the praises of fibre. Fibre is a complex carbohydrate that is not digested or absorbed by the body, so it doesn't provide us with energy like carbohydrates normally do. However, although it's not used as a source of energy, it offers us many other benefits, such as maintaining a healthy gut, supporting weight loss and lowering our risk of cardiovascular disease. Just 7g (about three to four servings of fruit and vegetables) of extra fibre a day can reduce the risk of CVD by 9 per cent. Considering CVD is one of the biggest causes of death in the UK and USA, this small reduction in risk could make a big impact on thousands of people.

Dietary fibre improves the risk of CVD in a number of ways:

1. Soluble fibre slows down the absorption of food from the gut, which reduces that big spike in blood glucose after a meal. This is particularly important for those with diabetes.

2. Reduces LDL (bad cholesterol) and total cholesterol. Although it remains unclear how this actually happens, it's believed to bind the cholesterol in the gut, reducing the amount absorbed.

3. Fibre adds volume to food slowing down the speed at which it passes through our gut, keeping us fuller longer, and also contributing to weight loss.

• Sodium

Sodium is naturally found in small quantities in most foods that we eat. The main source of sodium in our diet is sodium chloride, better known as salt.

We need some sodium in our diet as it helps control the fluid balance in our body, which influences our blood pressure. It acts on the kidneys to determine how much water we get rid of (i.e. how much we wee out) and how much to hold on to – so it is crucial for keeping us hydrated. This is why endurance athletes drink salt replacement drinks, such as Dioralyte after a long race.

This whole process is usually tightly regulated; however, excess sodium in the diet can tip the scale out of balance. The more salt we consume, the more water the body will try to hold on to. The extra fluid in the body pushes up the blood pressure, which puts strain on the heart and blood vessels. The walls thicken and narrow under the continued high pressure, and the heart is forced to pump harder to move blood around the body. Over time this can lead to serious health problems, such as stroke, kidney failure and heart disease.

The recommended amount of salt that we should have a day is 6g, which is about 2.4g of sodium; however, for most of us, that's a bit of an arbitrary number. What I would recommend is to not worry about the exact amount of salt that you eat but instead actively try to reduce the amount that you eat as much as possible.

If your diet is based on mostly processed foods, it's seriously easy to rack up that number. Let's compare a typical 'meal deal' shop-bought lunch with a home-made lunch and see how they compare.

As you can see, one meal alone made up of processed and packaged foods can total over half of your recommended sodium intake.

The majority of dietary sodium comes from processed foods, such as ready meals, tinned foods, processed meats, sauces, and even foods you wouldn't expect to contain high amounts of salt, such as cakes and biscuits – seriously, check the labels if you don't believe me. We can reduce the amount of salt that we have every day drastically by simply cutting out these foods

SHOP-BOUGHT LUNCH	SODIUM
BLT sandwich	930mg
1 packet of crisps	400mg
1 bottle of orange juice	12mg
	Total: 1,342mg

HOME-MADE LUNCH	SODIUM
Chicken breast, roasted butternut squash and broccoli	80mg
1 apple	0mg
1 bottle of water	6.5mg
	Total: 86.5mg

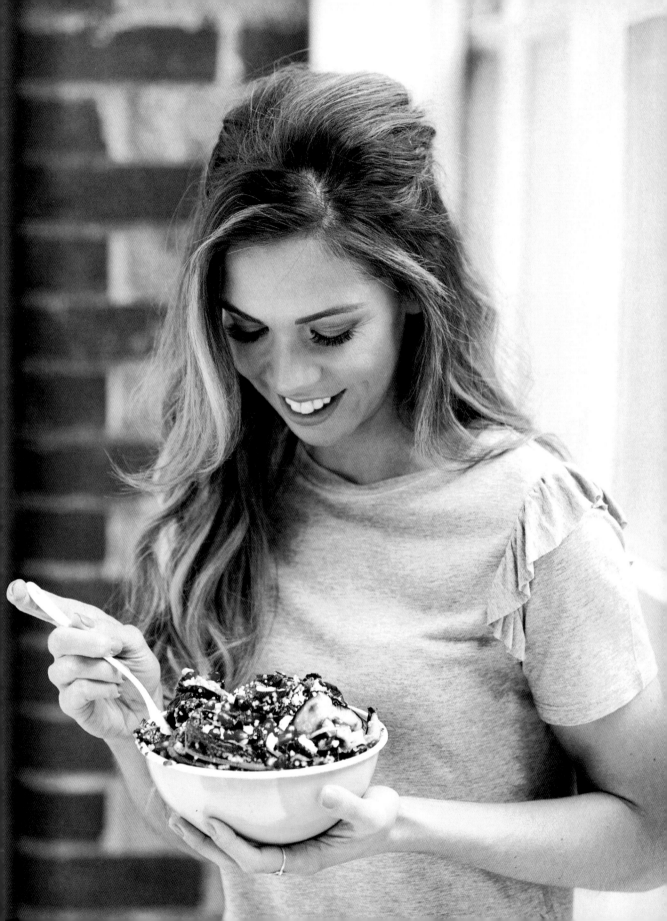

PHYSICAL ACTIVITY

Last, but certainly not least, physical exercise is one of the most important things we can do to improve our health, particularly our cardiovascular health. Regular exercise offers a number of health benefits which overall reduce the risk of cardiovascular disease:

- **Improves your level of fitness** – regular exercise forces the heart to pump blood faster around your body. To adapt to this increased workload, the muscle in the heart wall (known as the ventricular wall) increases in thickness so that it can pump blood more efficiently around the body.

- **Lower blood pressure** – in the short term, both blood pressure and heart rate increase during exercise to deliver more blood, and oxygen, to the muscles. You know that feeling when your heart is pounding in your chest and you can feel your blood rushing through your veins after you've sprinted? Yep, that's what I'm talking about. However, in the long-term, exercise decreases blood pressure by improving the elasticity of the blood vessels so that they can expand more easily and deliver oxygen to the muscles at a faster rate.

- **Improve cholesterol levels** – evidence shows that aerobic exercise can reduce the amount of bad (LDL) cholesterol and actually increase the amount of good (HDL) cholesterol.

- **Increase in insulin sensitivity** – insulin is the hormone that allows cells in the body to take up glucose, which is our main source of energy. People with diabetes, or insulin resistance, are not very sensitive to insulin so the glucose ends up hanging around in their bloodstream. Not only does this mean that the cells are starved of energy, but the excess sugar in the bloodstream travels around the body and over time causes damage to nerves and blood vessels. Regular exercise has been shown to improve insulin sensitivity, which helps the cells to take up the glucose that they need for energy.

- **Helps you maintain and lose extra weight** – countless studies show that obesity is a major risk factor for cardiovascular disease, and reducing the rates of obesity has become one of the biggest missions for public health authorities across the world. As doctors, we know the health implications of obesity and we know that weight loss can massively help reduce these risks. However, the sensitivity around the subject means that it's not always an easy subject to approach. Especially in light of 'body shaming' social media campaigns, weight loss advice can often be mistaken for 'fat-shaming'. The bottom line is: a person's body shape does not determine their health. We all have the genetic predisposition to be different shapes and sizes. However, if we are much heavier than a normal weight, or even much lighter, we run the risk of serious health problems that can reduce our life expectancy too. I've put together a Pick 'n' Mix workout plan, which I hope will inspire you (page 224).

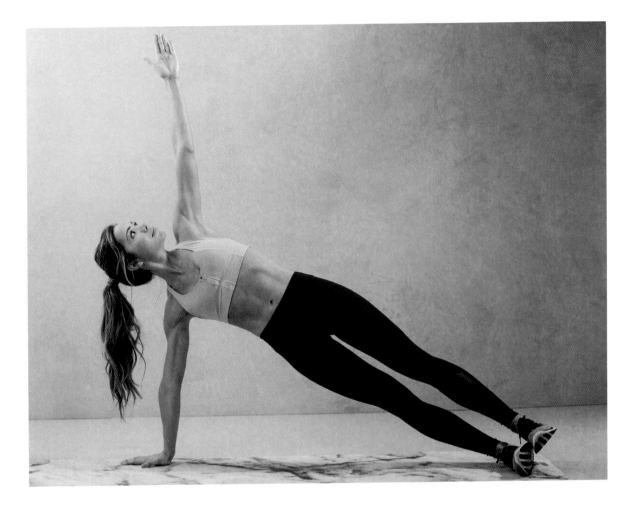

HEART-HEALTHY HEROES	SOURCES
OMEGA 3	Oily fish (*salmon, mackerel, sardines, tuna*), chia seeds, walnuts, hemp seeds
FIBRE	Wholegrains (*oats, wheat rye, brown rice, quinoa*), legumes (*lentils, beans and peas*), fruit and vegetables
LOW SODIUM	Unprocessed foods, seasoning with herbs and spices, home-made dressings and dips

THE BRAIN

Have you ever had 'butterflies in your tummy'? Or a really strong 'gut feeling' about something?

Our brain and gut are so closely linked that not only does our brain have an impact on our gut health, but our gut, and the food that we eat, massively influences our brain. This connection is known as the 'brain-gut axis' and it's one of the fastest-growing areas of research, in both the fields of medicine and nutrition. There is good evidence to suggest that our dietary habits massively influence brain health and mental function, and that poor nutrition is linked to a number of mental health conditions, such as anxiety and depression.

There is no evidence to suggest that food should completely replace medication in the treatment of mental health disorders, and this isn't something I would recommend, but I strongly believe that the right foods can be a very effective and beneficial part of the treatment plan. I've been there, and I've bought the T-shirt. When I was severely underweight, and my body and mind were stripped of the nutrients they so badly needed, my mood was at its lowest. I was so depressed that I found it too much of an effort to get out of bed, or to wash my hair, or to put a fork in my mouth. The day I hit rock bottom was the day I made the best decision of my life – to visit a dietician and use food to nourish me back to health.

Initially I didn't focus on eating healthily – but just eating full stop. I was scared of how malnourished I had become, particularly when my menstrual periods stopped and my hair began to thin and fall out. My blood results showed that I was very low in important nutrients, such as iron and calcium, and important sex hormones, FSH and LH, which regulate the menstrual cycle. Overwhelmed by the state I had left my body in, I promised myself that I would find a way back to health and happiness. I started to include more iron-rich foods in my diet, such as lean steak and dark green, leafy vegetables. I had a pot of Greek yogurt as a snack and a glass of milk with my breakfast every morning to increase my calcium intake. Despite my reluctance, my mum encouraged me to take cod liver oil supplements daily to boost my intake of healthy fats, which are essential for hormone production. Eating lots of really good food every day wasn't easy and there were many days when I wanted to throw in the towel. However, week by week, the more food I ate, and the more weight I put on, the more hopeful I became. I could think clearly again and focus on my future, something I had almost given up on. I began to actually enjoy eating, and enjoy cooking. My body grew stronger, my hair became thicker, my periods returned, and I started to laugh and smile again.

Our brain requires a lot of energy, and the right nutrients, to function correctly. Like every part of our body it requires rest, fresh air, adequate hydration, and good nutrition. There are some key nutrients in particular that are linked to brain health and performance:

- **HEALTHY FATS:
  omega 3 and omega 6**

My mum used to always tell me to eat fish the night before an exam for some 'brain food' and, although I didn't really understand why, I did it anyway – just in case. However, the idea that healthy fats can actually boost brain power and performance is no longer considered an old wives' tale.

Our brain requires a good balance of omega 3 and omega 6 polyunsaturated fatty acids (PUFAs) to function at its best. Omega 3 and omega 6 are essential fatty acids, which mean our bodies cannot make them and we need some help from our diet. The brain itself is made of 60 per cent fat and these special fatty acids make up an essential part of the covering of nerve cells. Not only do these fats play an important role in the make-up of nerve cells, but research shows that dietary intake of fatty acids has a role in brain performance and the prevention of mental health disorders, such as depression, and neurodegenerative disease, such as Alzheimer's.

As I said earlier, as well as being important that we get enough omega 3 and omega 6, it's important that we get the right balance of each. Omega 6 fatty acids promote inflammation and contribute to modern diseases, such as heart disease, obesity and diabetes. Although omega 6 is also an essential fatty acid, we unfortunately consume almost too much in the Western diet.

Omega 6 is found in vegetable and seed oils, and here in the Western world we can't seem to get enough of it. On average we consume ten to twenty times more of it compared to omega 3! I'm sure you're thinking that surely that must be a good thing? Well, all of this excess omega 6 means our bodies are in an inflamed state, which makes us more likely to develop the so-called 'inflammatory' diseases like inflammatory bowel disease, autoimmune diseases, and Alzheimer's disease. So although omega 6 is an essential fatty acid, we need much less of it than we need omega 3 so focus on getting most of your essential fatty acids from omega 3-rich sources, such as oily fish, like salmon and mackerel, avocados, flaxseed and walnuts.

- **Vitamin D**

Who doesn't feel instantly cheerful when it's a beautiful, sunny day out? Part of that reason may be because you can picnic outside, chill in the park, or simply walk to work, but one major factor is our friend vitamin D – aka the sunshine vitamin. Vitamin D is unique because it is made in the body following exposure of the skin to sunlight. Many of us link winter blues with the lack of sunshine, so it's no surprise that low vitamin D has been linked to depression and other mood disorders. To guard against this, I take a Vitamin D supplement during the winter months. Vitamin D receptors can be found in many important areas of the brain and as a result vitamin D plays an important role in brain function and development. Our main source of vitamin D production is sunlight, but for those of us living further away from the equator, this is why it's so important that we get a little extra through our diet. Many foods, such as breakfast cereals, bread and milk are fortified with vitamin D nowadays so deficiency is less common. However, as they are artificially fortified, it's likely that they've undergone other forms of processing to get to the end product. My recommendation would be to not depend on the fortified foods, and instead opt for natural sources, such as oily fish, yogurt and cheese.

• Vitamin B12 and folate

Vitamin B12 is involved in the metabolism of all cells and works with folate to make DNA and red blood cells. Vitamin B12 also plays a major role in the nervous system and helps produce the fatty insulation that wraps around our nerves, helping to transmit messages from one part of our body to another. All of the B vitamins, particularly B12, are essential for the formation of chemicals in the brain, called neurotransmitters, which affect mood and support healthy functioning of the nervous system.

Pregnant women are recommended to take folate supplements on top of their diet, as it is essential for the development of the baby's brain and spinal cord. However, this vitamin isn't just essential during the foetal period but also throughout life. Vitamin B12 and folate deficiency is usually only picked up when people become anaemic, i.e. they have fewer red blood cells than normal or have too little haemoglobin in each red blood cell. Anaemia usually presents as fatigue or lack of energy, but more severe, chronic deficiencies of vitamin B12 can lead to mouth ulcers, muscle weakness, pins and needles, and neurological problems.

Vitamin B12 is found only in animal foods, such as red meat, eggs and shellfish, or plant foods that are fortified. Vegans can become deficient in this vitamin very easily so it's important to opt for fortified products or vitamin B12 supplementation if you exclude animal products from your diet. Folate is found in lentils and leafy green vegetables – think folate = foliage = green plant foods.

• Probiotics

Our gut is often referred to as our second brain as our mood is intimately linked to the function of our digestive system. The gut microbiome refers to all bacteria living inside our gut – the good and the bad. When there is an imbalance between the beneficial bacteria in the gut and disease-causing bacteria, our physical health can be jeopardised leading to digestive problems, such as irritable bowel syndrome (IBS). However, a disruption in the gut flora has also been associated with mental health conditions, such as anxiety and depression. I try to include plenty of probiotic and prebiotic foods in my diet.

There are a number of things that can disrupt the balance of good and bad bacteria in the gut, such as long-term antibiotic use, alcohol, stress and a poor diet. However, the good news is that we can heal our gut and restore the harmony between our gut bacteria.

There is a lot of new evidence suggesting that probiotic supplementation can improve mood and feelings of anxiety, acting as a potential adjuvant in the treatment of depression. It's important for me to highlight that medication, particularly antidepressants, can be essential for some people and that I do not recommend replacing them with food. However, regardless of whether you suffer from low mood or not, probiotics are a safe way to nourish and support the growth of our good bacteria.

Probiotics are live cultures of bacteria and you probably eat some form of probiotic on a daily basis. I get most of my intake through Greek yogurt but I also add pickled foods like gherkins and red cabbage to my salads – yep, I'm that person at the table who will eat the unwanted pickles from everyone's burger!

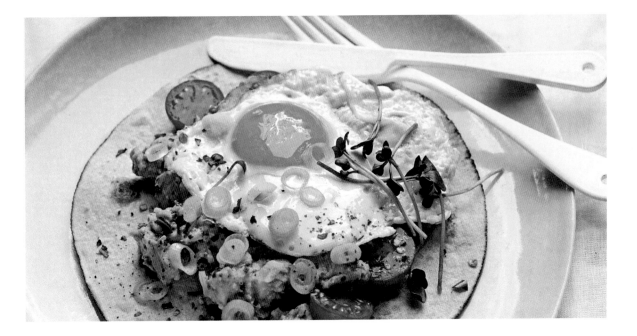

GOOD MOOD FOODS	SOURCES
OMEGA 3	Mackerel, salmon, walnuts, brazil nuts, chia seeds, sardines, hemp seeds, egg yolks, cod liver oil
VITAMIN D	Sunshine, fortified cereals and breads, salmon, tuna, mackerel, cheese, eggs
VITAMIN B12	Red meat, salmon, cod, milk, cheese, eggs
FOLATE	Broccoli, kale, spinach, asparagus, chickpeas, beans and lentils
PROBIOTICS	Natural yogurt, cottage cheese, sauerkraut, tempeh, kefir

THE DIGESTIVE SYSTEM

It's no wonder that a healthy digestive system is the cornerstone to overall health and well-being – our digestive system is responsible for the breakdown of food, removal of waste products, absorption of nutrients, and defence against harmful bugs and toxins. If digestion is compromised for any reason, whether it is due to poor diet, stress or disease, this can totally disrupt absorption of important nutrients and also cause unpleasant symptoms, such as bloating, diarrhoea and wind.

Irritable bowel syndrome (IBS) is one of the most common gut problems affecting 10–20 per cent of us in the UK – and that's just including those who have been officially diagnosed. How is IBS diagnosed? In medicine it's known as a 'diagnosis of exclusion'. This means that it's a label given when other conditions, such as inflammatory bowel disease (Crohn's disease and ulcerative colitis) and coeliac disease are ruled out. The difficulty with a condition like IBS is that it cannot be diagnosed by a simple blood test which means that a lot of people self-diagnose. This can be really dangerous as the symptoms of IBS are also symptoms of other conditions or diseases, some of which are much more sinister than IBS. On the flip side, it can also be a false diagnosis when there is no real, underlying condition. Many people diagnose themselves with IBS because the symptoms are so vague that it is pretty easy to convince yourself that you have it – bloating, diarrhoea and flatulence? I'm sure many of us suffer after an Indian curry. This is why it is so important to talk to your GP if you think that you may have IBS, or any condition for that matter. With so much information at our fingertips it is far too easy to fall into the trap of diagnosing online. I've touched on this before when I discussed one of the self-diagnoses du jour – gluten intolerance!

Regardless of having the diagnosis of IBS, the majority of us at some point in our lives will go through periods where our gut isn't functioning quite as well as it should be. This can be down to a number of things from the foods that we're eating, medications we're taking, and the stress we're undergoing in our lives. I'm sure you can relate to this the night before a big event, like an exam, when you're running back and forth to the loo with an upset tummy.

A healthy gut depends on lots of things that are out of our control, like disease and stress, but one thing which we can control is the food that we eat, and certain foods are absolutely key in achieving a healthy gut.

• Probiotics & prebiotics

Probiotics, that old chestnut again. As horrible as it may sound, the gut is home to over 500 different species of bacteria. We grow up learning that bacteria is bad news: it causes infections, gives us coughs and colds, and spoils our food. Of course this is true but not all bacteria cause us health problems, some bacteria actually does us a lot of good. Friendly bacteria in our gut, such as lactobacillus and bifidobacteria, are essential for a strong immune system and overall health. These bacteria support us by: fending off disease-causing bacteria, producing vitamins, including vitamin K, and helping us digest insoluble fibre, such as starch and cellulose. Certain foods naturally contain good bacteria, such as natural yogurt and cottage cheese, but you can also pick up fortified drinks in the supermarket.

While probiotics introduce good bacteria into the gut, prebiotics act as a food source, or a fertiliser, for the good bacteria. They help the good bacteria to survive and thrive in the gut. Prebiotics are insoluble fibres, which mainly come from the outer parts of fruit and vegetables, wholegrains and legumes.

• Fibre

As we discussed earlier, dietary fibre is a non-digestible carbohydrate, which means we cannot break it down and use if for energy. Although it offers us little in the way of energy, it encourages digestion and absorption of other food so it is essential for good gut health. There are two main types of fibre: soluble and insoluble. Insoluble fibre helps to bulk up stools and to maintain bowel regularity. This type of fibre is found in wholegrains, flaxseed, fruit and vegetables.

Soluble fibre includes pectins and gums, which form a gel when mixed with liquid. Soluble fibre is a prebiotic which is fermented by our healthy gut bacteria. As we know, not only is this fibre important for our gut health but has also been linked to improved cardiovascular health, lower levels of cholesterol, and improved blood sugar control. Soluble fibre is found in wholegrains, such as oats and brown rice, beans and lentils, and fruit and vegetables.

Don't forget, if you're not accustomed to having much fibre in your diet, increase your intake slowly by 2–3g (about the amount of fibre in an apple) and see how you feel. Some people can be very sensitive to increases in fibre and may find that they experience some bloating initially.

• Rest and digest

When we are making a conscious effort to live healthier lives we automatically focus on our diet and physical health, and often neglect our mental health. Stress is often the reason why people still suffer from problems with their gut, despite following a healthy diet.

The majority of us have very busy lives and are constantly stressed as a result. Studies consistently show that people with anxiety, depression and other mood disorders are far more likely to have digestive problems and vice versa. Stress affects the gut in several different ways. Stress speeds up the passage of food and stools through the intestine, which can lead to diarrhoea, and impair absorption of water and important nutrients.

As I've mentioned before, the gut really is an important part of the nervous system.

A key component of a healthy lifestyle should include stress management techniques.

The intestine has its own network of nerves known as the enteric system, which is influenced by signalling from the brain. One way to understand this is the nausea we feel when we are anxious or excited about something.

Relaxing is easier said than done and for most of us, it's difficult to switch off from the external stressors in our lives, such as work and finance. That said, it goes without saying that a key component of a healthy lifestyle should include stress management techniques. In current practice, the first line of treatment for most mental health conditions, such as mild depression is non-pharmacological interventions, such as 'talk therapy', mindfulness and exercise. I first tried mindfulness during my psychiatry rotation as a medical student. Within the group of patients attending the class, there was no one person with the same mental health disorder; the conditions ranged from obsessive compulsive disorder to anorexia, but they were all attending the same type of therapy – mindfulness. Those patients voluntarily attended the weekly sessions, and would share with one another the new milestones that they had made with their individual conditions.

Whether it's mindfulness and meditation that helps you unwind, or something as simple as going for a ten-minute walk in the evening, whatever it is – do it. The benefits of stress management reach far beyond a healthy gut, but our mental health is something we tend to neglect when it comes to approaching our health.

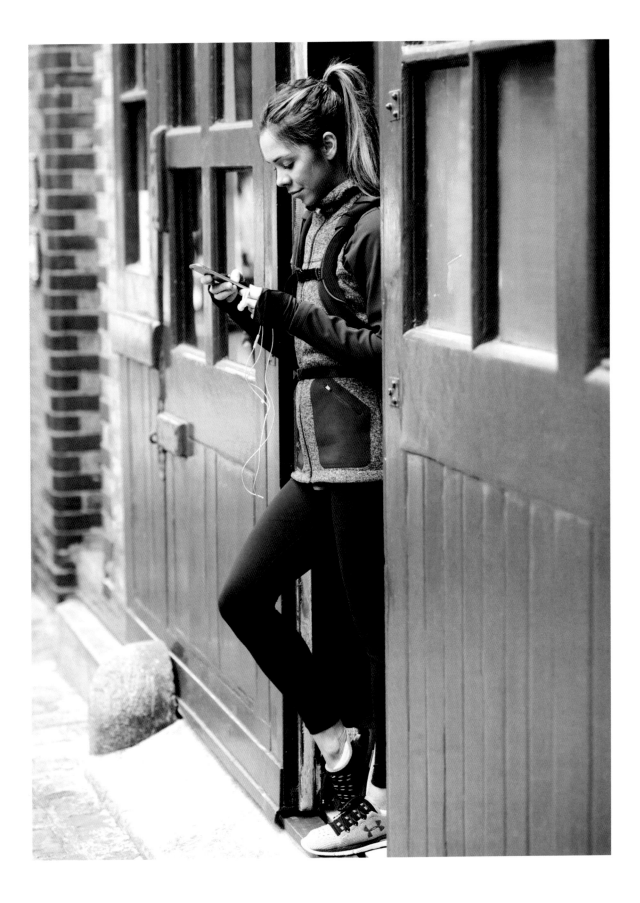

GUT HINDERING

During my first year at university, I started to suffer from IBS-like symptoms of bloating, tummy pain, and alternating bouts of diarrhoea and constipation. I put it down to the stress I was under but my GP suggested that I keep a food diary and see if anything made it worse. Everything seemed to flare it up, but 90 per cent of my food was based around refined grains and processed foods containing wheat, such as bread, pasta and bowls of sugary cereal. It wasn't until I actually wrote down what I was eating that I realised how lazy I had become with my diet. I took it upon myself to cut those foods out to see what would happen, and I increased my intake of fruit and vegetables to make up for it. I lost weight, my energy levels increased, my skin was clearer, I was less bloated and my digestive problems began to settle.

I can't prove that the reason I felt better was because I cut out these wheat-containing foods, or if I simply felt better because I cut down on processed foods and started eating real, whole foods. What I do know, however, is that making those dietary changes made a positive impact on my health.

Since then I've reintroduced some gluten into my diet in very small amounts. I now eat oats and rye bread without any issues, but when I have eaten anything with wheat flour, such as bread, my digestive issues flare back up. I guess you can say I've experimented with myself over the past few years, and I know which foods fuel me well and make me feel great. There are certain foods I can tolerate in small amounts, such as dairy and whey protein, but too much in one day causes me a lot of discomfort. Although I don't recommend using yourself as a guinea pig, I do recommend listening to your body and being mindful of those foods that make you feel great and those that do not.

If you are struggling with bloating and cramping, keeping a food diary and narrowing down the foods that don't seem to agree with you is a good place to start. Foods that trigger these uncomfortable symptoms can differ from one person to the next but there are some notorious culprits that are often to blame, such as:

- **Sugar alcohol & sweeteners**

Sugar alcohols, such as xylitol and erythritol, are used as a lower calorie substitute for sugar in low-cal and low-sugar foods. Scan the label of any 'diet' product on the shelves and I'm sure you will find at least one of these sugar alcohols in the list of ingredients (amongst many other weird and wonderful chemicals). They contain fewer calories than table sugar and natural sweeteners, like honey and maple syrup, and are less likely to spike our blood sugar levels. On the whole, they are considered safe and relatively healthy, and can actually be a very useful dietary sugar substitute for those with diabetes or those trying to lose weight. The issue is that they are really hard to digest, so our gut bacteria have to do most of the hard work for us. If we consume too much of this stuff, all this fermentation by our gut bacteria can lead to gas, bloating and diarrhoea.

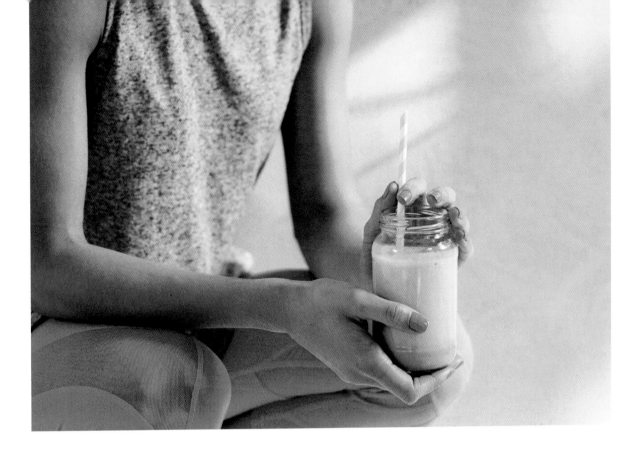

• Soft drinks

The reason soda, or soft drinks, are bubbly is because of a gas called carbonic acid. It's a very weak acid and isn't harmful, but it can lead to a build-up of air in the stomach which leads to bloating, burping and flatulence. If you already have underlying digestive problems, like IBS, soft drinks can aggravate them and worsen the symptoms. On top of this, soft drinks are usually packed with sweeteners and caffeine which tend to produce laxative effects. Try swapping your fizzy pop for plain old H20. If you find it difficult to drink tap water, try adding lemon, cucumber or mint to make it easier to sip on.

• Refined grains

Refined grains include white bread, white pasta, white rice and baked goods made with white flour. The reason they are white is because during processing the outer bran and germ layers are removed. Most of the fibre, vitamins and minerals are stored in these layers so our end product is a starchy carbohydrate which is low in nutrients. We don't have to work as hard to digest refined grains because most of it was done in the factory for us. This means the carbohydrates are digested and absorbed, and the sugar is quickly shuttled into our bloodstream. This can cause our blood-sugar levels to spike and then quickly crash, leaving us drained of energy. The lack of fibre can cause our gut to become sluggish and lazy, leading to constipation and haemorrhoids.

• Caffeine

If you find that your morning coffee is shortly followed by a timely bowel movement, you're not alone. Caffeine is a bowel stimulant, and what this means is that it essentially causes the muscles in the gut wall to contract and relax – a process called peristalsis. A strong cup of coffee is often the perfect trick to help keep things moving. However, the faster movement of food through our gut means that less water is absorbed leading to looser stools. So before you order that grande triple shot Americano, be warned – excessive caffeine consumption can cause abdominal pain and diarrhoea.

• Processed foods

Processed foods are manufactured in such a way that they are often very quick and easy to eat. The texture is usually soft because most of the fibre is removed. This means we can eat more in a shorter amount of time, but we also use less energy (and burn fewer calories) digesting them than we would if they were unprocessed whole foods. Take a slice of white bread and compare it to a slice of seeded rye bread. The white bread almost dissolves in your mouth before you even begin to nibble it, but the rye bread requires a substantial amount of chewing, which means it takes a lot more time and effort to eat. This not only forces you to savour your meal, but it gives your brain time to realise it's full so you're less likely to overeat. All that extra fibre adds volume to the meal which further fills you up. Not to forget that processed foods are also laden with preservatives, additives and other chemicals that our bodies are not designed to deal with. We can cut down on this chemical storm by eating more wholesome, real foods.

GUT HEALING	GUT HINDERING
Natural yogurt	Low sugar or diet foods
Cottage cheese	Soft drinks
Sauerkraut	Coffee and other
Tempeh	caffeinated drinks
Bananas	White bread
Flax	White rice
Quinoa	White pasta
Oats	Processed foods
Brown rice	Takeaways

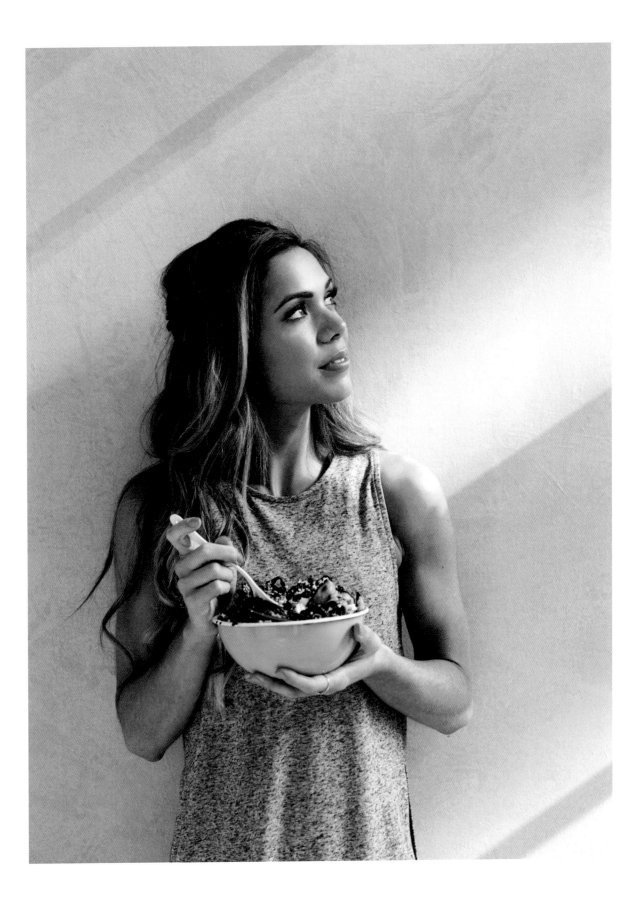

HAIR, SKIN AND NAILS

We all know that the food we eat has a huge impact on how our body looks and feels, but we often forget about the impact our diet has on our skin.

Many of my family members suffer from psoriasis, which is a common skin condition that causes red, flaky, crusty patches of inflamed skin. I fortunately do not have psoriasis but I've always had quite dry skin. When I was very underweight, my skin was so dry that it would often crack and cause me pain and itching. I would sit in front of the TV before bed at night applying moisturiser to my feet and then sleep in socks to help soothe the itching caused by the cracked skin. My once thick and glossy hair also dried out and became thin and lifeless.

Although my skin now is far from perfect, it's certainly the best it's ever been. I don't need to use emollients or intensive moisturisers any longer, and I often receive compliments on how good my skin looks and how bright my eyes are. I still believe that looking after your skin with a good skincare routine is important, but I'm not the type of girl who spends a lot of money on her face cream. The food that we eat affects every organ in our body, and we often forget that our skin is the largest organ in the body and our first line of defence. Before we start worrying about what we are putting onto our skin, we should be thinking about what we are putting into our bodies – and into our skin.

Any good diet will work wonders for our skin regardless of what food we eat, but there are a number of vitamins and minerals that are key to glowing skin:

- **Vitamin A**

Vitamin A is an antioxidant that helps to protect cells against free radicals and UV damage, and reduce the signs of ageing. This vitamin is essential for cell renewal and repair and as it promotes cell turnover, it helps to keep the skin smooth and soft, and prevents the blockage of skin pores. Deficiency of vitamin A can lead to dry, scaly skin and a condition known as hyperkeratosis pillaris, which appears as raised, reddened bumps around hair follicles on the back of the arms. The active form of vitamin A is known as retinol. Synthetic retinoids are often used by dermatologists in the treatment of certain skin conditions, such as psoriasis and acne. However, we can find vitamin A naturally in a variety of foods, particularly cod liver oil, egg yolks, and dairy.

During pregnancy, vitamin A intake should be reduced as an excess can be harmful to the developing baby.

- **Vitamin C**

Vitamin C is another powerful antioxidant, protecting our skin against environmental damage and preventing signs of ageing. Vitamin C plays an essential role in the production of collagen, a structural protein in our skin that maintains the skin's strength and elasticity. Vitamin C deficiency, known as scurvy, is uncommon nowadays, particularly in developed countries. Symptoms of scurvy are a result of impaired collagen production which present as bleeding gums, poor wound healing and loss of teeth. Although we may not be at risk of scurvy, observational studies have shown that increasing the amount of vitamin C in the diet can improve skin appearance and reduce the signs of ageing. Vitamin C is abundant in colourful fruit and vegetables so aim to load up on these beauty foods on a regular basis.

Vitamin C is heat-sensitive, so snack on raw veggies to get the greatest benefit.

• Vitamin E

Vitamin E is another one of our superhero antioxidants, protecting our skin against the damaging effects of the environment. Adequate levels of this vitamin in the skin may help to reduce the effects of ageing and reduce the risk of skin cancer. Vitamin E can be found on our skin and is secreted here through the oil in our skin: sebum. It is also found in many cosmetic skincare products as it can be absorbed topically also. Foods rich in vitamin E include nuts, seeds and olive oil.

• Omega 3

Healthy fats, particularly the omega 3 fatty acids, are essential for glowing skin, and strong hair and nails. Omega 3 and omega 6 are both essential fatty acids that we need to obtain from our diet. As I mentioned earlier, the modern diet tends to have far too much omega 6 (pro-inflammatory) and not enough omega 3 (anti-inflammatory). This high ratio of omega 6 to omega 3 has been linked to an increase in the prevalence of inflammatory skin conditions, such as acne and psoriasis. Increasing our dietary intake of omega 3 can reduce the redness, scaling and itching caused by these skin conditions, and can also aid in the appearance of smoother, younger-looking skin.

• Zinc

Zinc is an essential trace element. It plays a number of important roles in the body from supporting the body's immune system, hormone production and fertility, and the formation of important proteins. In skin, this mineral assists in wound healing, reducing inflammation and protection against UV damage. Zinc is also essential for normal function of the oil-producing glands in our skin, known as sebaceous glands, which help to keep skin and hair moisturised and strong. Symptoms of zinc deficiency range from hair loss, brittle nails, impaired wound healing and decreased fertility.

TIP: *Zinc is best absorbed from animal sources, as plant-based sources, such as fibrous fruit, vegetables and grains, contain a mineral called phytic acid. Phytic acid can bind to important micronutrients, such as iron and zinc and impair their absorption into the body. It is possible to reduce the effects of phytic acid in plant-based foods by soaking and cooking the foods first. If you're not vegan or vegetarian, opt for shellfish and red meat for the best zinc sources.*

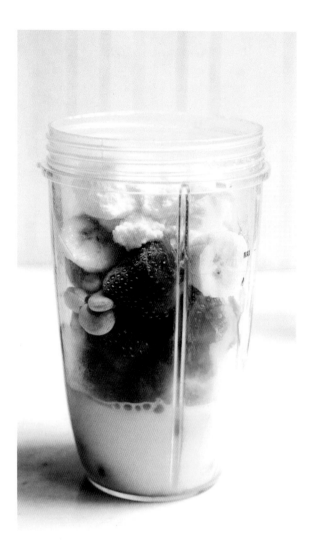

Any good diet will work wonders for you and your skin regardless of what food you eat.

• Selenium

Selenium is another essential mineral and powerful antioxidant. This mineral acts as a co-factor to an important detoxifying enzyme known as glutathione peroxidase. It can therefore help to reduce inflammation, premature aging and skin cancer, caused by free radicals. Selenium also has a role in skin elasticity and maintaining its youthful appearance. Vitamin E and selenium complement one another, so pair them together for added benefit. Brazil nuts are the best-known sources of selenium – just two a day provide you with your recommended daily allowance.

• Silica

Silica is less well known than the other minerals but it is certainly just as important, particularly for skin health. Silica plays an important role in the formation of collagen which helps to keep skin smooth and firm. Deficiency can lead to weak hair, nails and skin, and impaired wound healing. Silica is found in the soil, and the best sources of this mineral are raw organic fruit and vegetables.

• Niacin (vitamin B3)

Niacin, or vitamin B3, deficiency leads to a condition known as 'pellagra' with symptoms known as the four Ds: diarrhoea, dementia, dermatitis and death (if left untreated). Sounds nasty? It is, but thankfully pellagra hasn't been an issue since the seventeenth or eighteenth century. However, the skin conditions, such as dermatitis, which occur as a result of the deficiency highlight the important role that niacin has in skin health. In fact, the word 'pellagra' comes from 'pelle agra', the Italian phrase for rough skin. Although niacin deficiency is rare in healthy individuals, some conditions, such as coeliac disease and IBS may reduce the absorption of the vitamin. The best sources of niacin include poultry, fish, legumes and cereals.

• Water

We have all been told time and time again that we should be drinking six to eight glasses of water a day, but what benefit has this on our skin? Almost 60 per cent of your skin is made up of water and functions as a protective barrier to prevent excess fluid loss. Adequate hydration helps to moisturise dry skin in addition to improving the appearance of fine lines and wrinkles. To keep your skin's natural glow, make sure to moisture daily to lock in that hydration.

SKIN-SAVING NUTRIENTS	BEST SOURCE
Vitamin A	Liver, cod liver oil, egg yolks, butter, pumpkins, carrots, kale and spinach
Vitamin C	Citrus fruits, kiwis, melons, berries, papayas, bell peppers, broccoli and cabbages
Vitamin E	Almonds, avocados, olives, olive oil, sunflower seeds, egg yolks and spinach
Zinc	Liver, oysters, shellfish, red meat, eggs, chia seeds, chickpeas and quinoa
Omega 3	Salmon, sardines, tuna, trout, flaxseeds, walnuts and chia seeds
Selenium	Brazil nuts, tuna, shellfish and mushrooms
Silica	Leeks, cucumbers, asparagus, celery, strawberries, chickpeas and rhubarb
Niacin	Turkey, chicken, tuna, salmon, beef, fortified cereals, legumes and milk

SHOPPING LIST

MEAT, POULTRY + FISH
- Free-range eggs
- Lean steak mince
- Chicken breasts (*free-range where possible*)
- Chicken mince
- Grass-fed steaks
- Salmon fillets
- Smoked salmon
- Cod fillets

DAIRY + DAIRY-FREE ALTERNATIVES
- Greek yogurt
- Coconut yogurt (*DF*)
- Unsweetened almond milk (*DF*)
- Feta
- Halloumi
- Quark

OILS + FATS
- Grass-fed butter
- Extra-virgin coconut oil
- Extra-virgin olive oil

NUTS + SEEDS
- Almond butter
- Peanut butter
- Almonds
- Cashews
- Hazelnuts
- Pine nuts
- Brazil nuts
- Chia seeds
- Sesame seeds
- Flaxseeds

WHOLEGRAIN + PULSES
- Oats (*GF if necessary*)
- Brown rice
- Quinoa
- Puy lentils
- Red kidney beans
- Black beans
- Chickpeas
- Rye bread
- Rice cakes

HERBS, SPICES + SEASONING
- Basil
- Black pepper
- Smoked paprika
- Garlic
- Onions
- Oregano
- Turmeric
- Cinnamon
- Nutmeg
- Dill
- Chilli powder
- Cayenne pepper
- Rosemary
- Mint
- Soy sauce or tamari (GF)
- Sea salt
- Tahini
- Balsamic vinegar
- White wine vinegar
- Wholegrain mustard
- Dijon mustard
- Fresh chillis

BAKING ESSENTIALS
- Coconut flour
- Ground almonds
- Baking powder
- Bicarbonate of soda
- Stevia
- Raw honey
- Desiccated coconut
- Cacao or cocoa powder
- Cacao nibs

FRUIT
- Strawberries
- Blueberries
- Raspberries
- Apples
- Bananas
- Lemons
- Limes
- Avocados
- Dates
- Goji berries
- Raisins

VEGETABLES
- Kale
- Spinach
- Courgettes
- Tomatoes
- Red onions
- Butternut squash
- Sweet potatoes
- Frozen peas
- Mixed bell peppers
- Carrots
- Broccoli
- Aubergines
- Cauliflowers
- Mixed lettuce leaves
- Mushrooms
- Beetroots

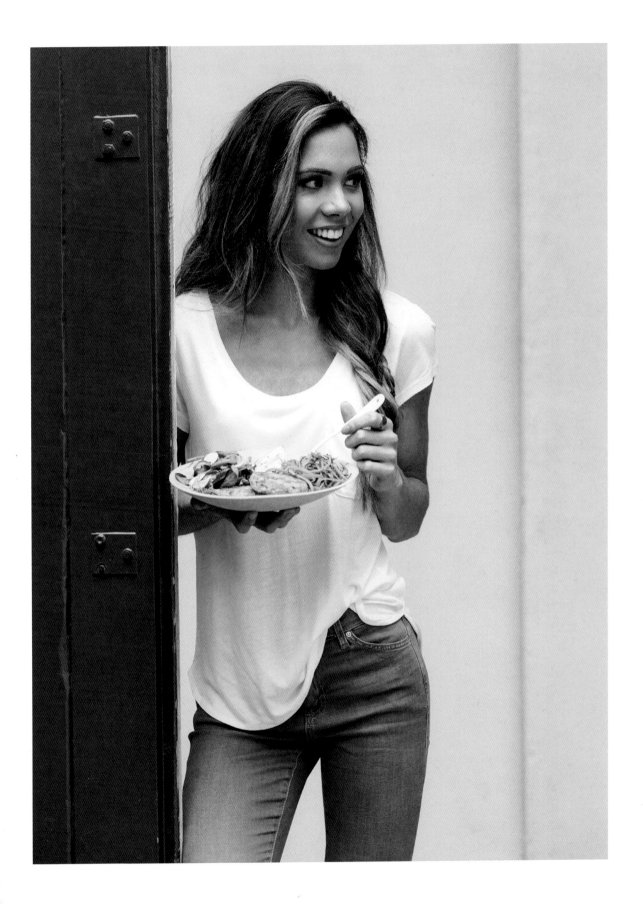

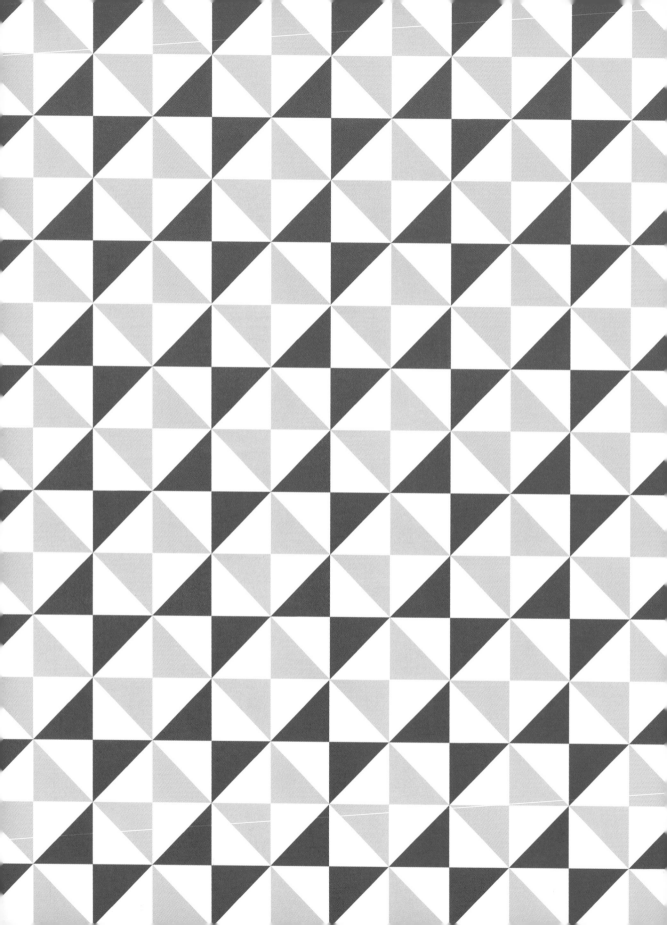

BREAKFAST

Breakfast is most definitely my favourite meal of the day.

Growing up, I was always told never to leave the house without a good breakfast and now as an adult, I still stick to this rule. If I'm starting my day exceptionally early, I usually grab a shake or smoothie (pages 110–127) to take with me on-the-go or I will pre-prepare some chocolate and banana overnight protein oats (page 98) or boil some eggs the day before to smash on rye toast (page 100) when I get to work.

In the summer, I usually crave cold, fresh breakfasts like smoothie bowls (page 84) and my superhero bircher muesli (page 92) and then when the colder months start to roll in, I look forward to a warm bowl of baked banana and chia spiced oatmeal (page 86). If I fancy something savoury, then sweet potato and chorizo hash with baked eggs (page 102) is always a good idea!

A lot of my breakfast recipes include oats – remember to use the gluten-free variety if you are intolerant to gluten.

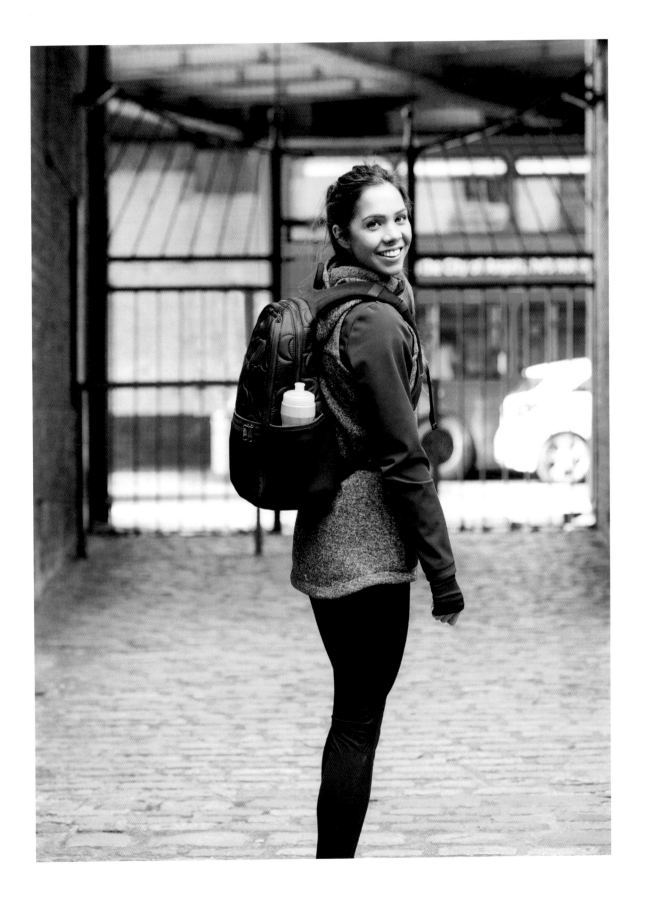

CHOCOLATE HAZELNUT PROTEIN OATS

Dessert for breakfast? Erm, yes please! If you're like me and love something sweet for breakfast, this chocolately, nutty protein oatmeal recipe is the perfect cure for any sugar craving. Not only does it taste amazing, but it is also low in sugar, high in fibre and packed full of protein.

SERVES 1

50g oats
1 tbsp cacao or cocoa powder
250ml almond milk or water
1 tbsp chocolate protein powder
Handful of hazelnuts, roughly
    chopped
1 square of 85 per cent dark
    chocolate, grated

Combine the oats and cacao powder in a microwaveable bowl and then pour in the milk or water. Microwave for 2–3 minutes until cooked. Stir.

Add the protein powder and stir well, adding more milk or water if necessary.

Sprinkle the chopped nuts and grated chocolate on top before serving.

PS... The protein powder may be omitted entirely or substituted with extra cacao powder; though it will become less protein-rich.

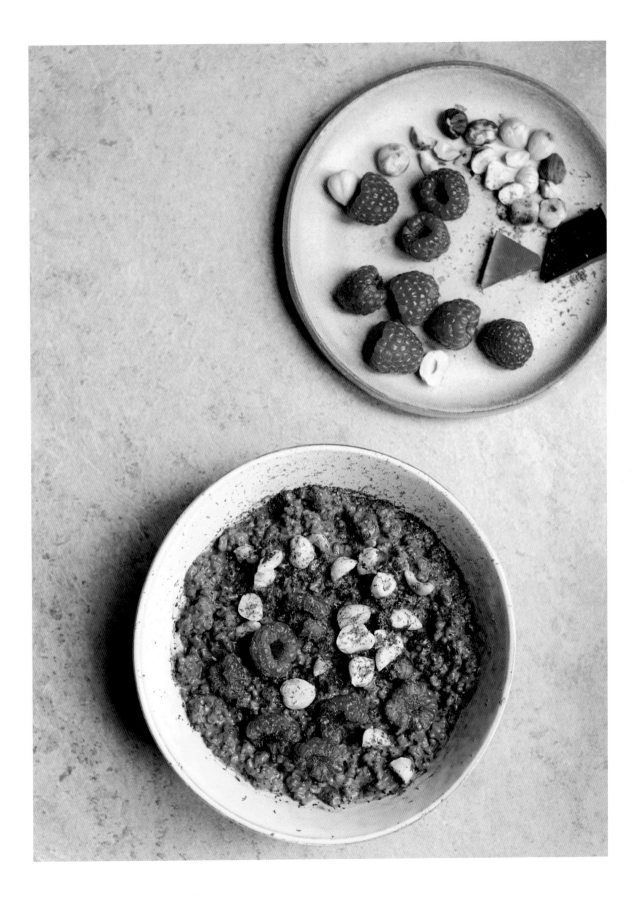

SUPERFOOD SMOOTHIE BOWL

You've probably noticed that smoothie bowls are dominating your Instagram feed lately – and for good reason! Not only do they look incredible, but they're packed full of good stuff too – leafy greens full of vitamins and minerals, creamy avocado crammed with healthy fats, and nutrient-packed fruits. The consistency is a lot thicker than a smoothie, so it's much more filling and almost ice cream-like.

SERVES 1

1 x 170g of tub Greek yogurt
½ ripe avocado
1 frozen banana
Handful of ice cubes
100ml almond milk
1 tbsp Stevia or sweetener
  (*optional*)
1 tsp vanilla essence
1 tsp matcha powder

SUGGESTED TOPPINGS
Nuts, seeds, fresh fruit, dried fruit, coconut, nut butter, agave nectar (a vegan alternative to honey), bee pollen

Blend all of the ingredients together in a food processor or blender and pour into a bowl.

Top with fruits, nuts, seeds or anything else that takes your fancy.

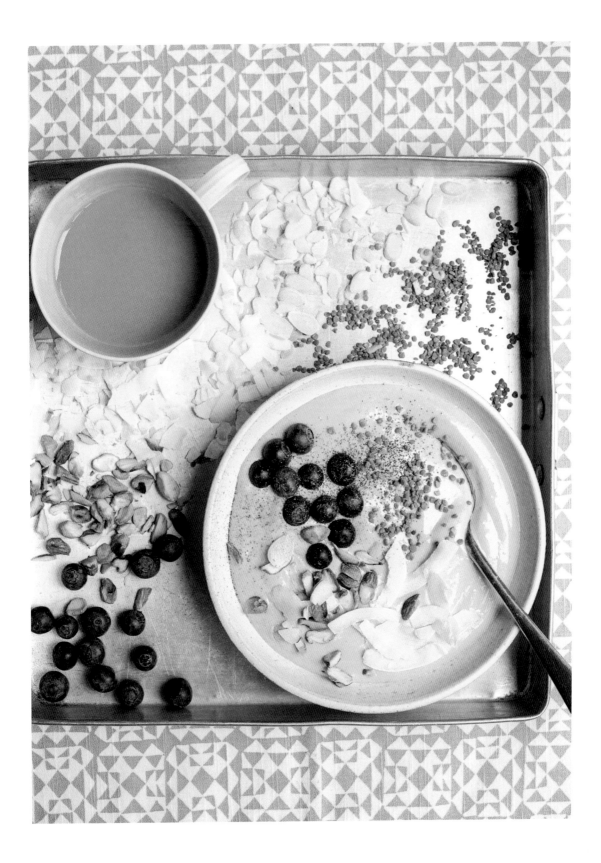

BAKED BANANA + CHIA SPICED OATMEAL

If you're a fan of banana bread, then this is the breakfast of dreams! Banana turns it from a regular bowl of porridge to a warm, fluffy cake for one. However, if you're short on time, you can cook it fully in the microwave for 2–3 minutes and skip the oven. It's totally delicious either way.

SERVES 1

1 banana, sliced lengthways
50g oats
30g protein powder
200–250ml almond milk
1 tbsp raisins
1 tbsp chia seeds
1 tsp cinnamon
1 tsp nutmeg

Preheat the oven to 180°C/350°F/gas mark 4.

Mash half the banana and set the other half aside.

Combine the mashed banana with the oats, protein, almond milk, raisins, chia seeds, cinnamon and nutmeg. Stir well.

Microwave the mixture on full for 2–3 minutes and stir again.

Transfer the mixture to an ovenproof bowl. Sprinkle over the fruit and seed mix, and place the other half of the banana on top. Bake for 25–30 minutes.

Remove from the oven and allow it to cool for 10 minutes before tucking in.

PS... The protein powder can be omitted, just reduce the amount of milk accordingly.

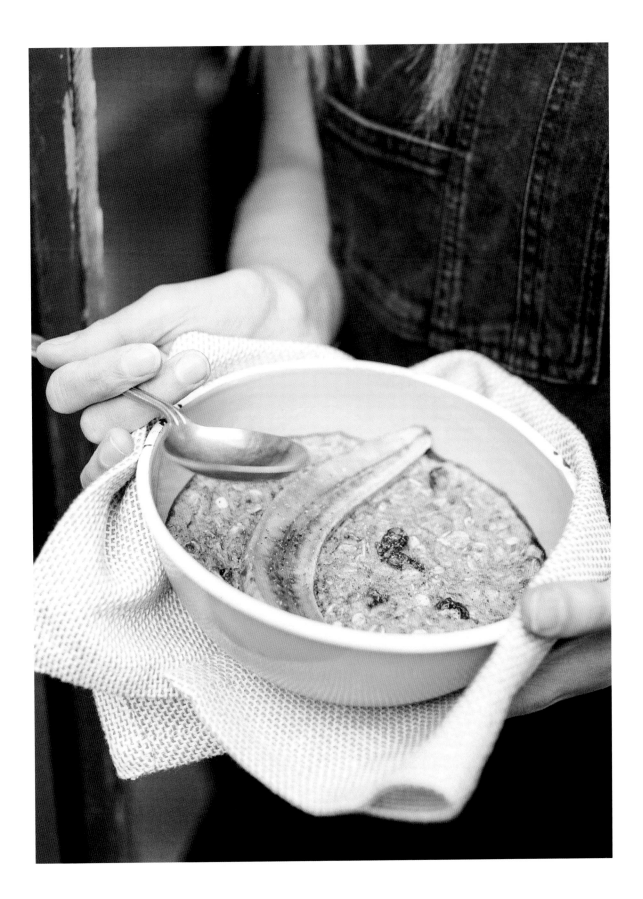

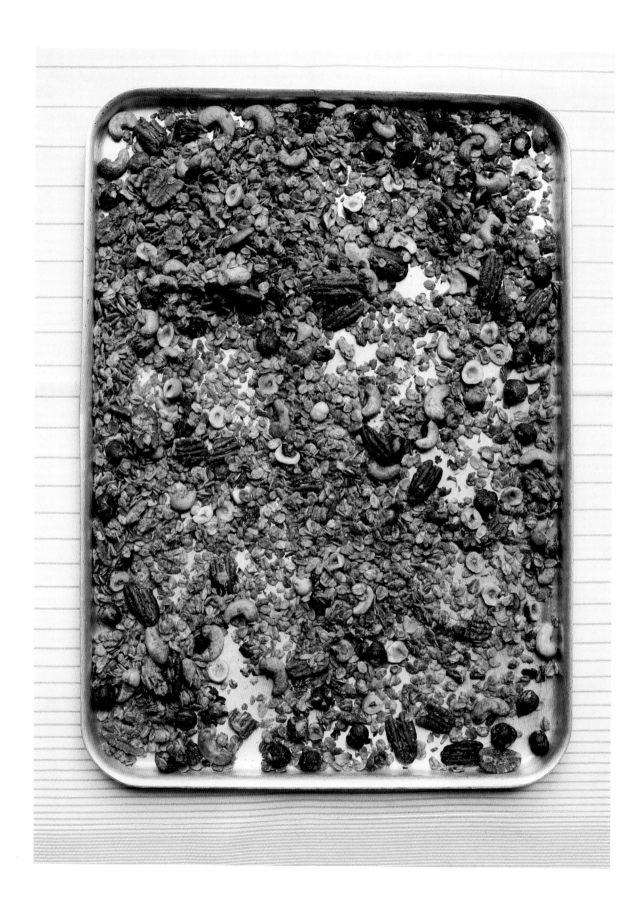

LOWER-SUGAR NUTTY CINNAMON GRANOLA

Most shop-bought granolas are alarmingly high in refined sugar – which is why it's so hard to stop at a couple of spoonfuls. I've got good news and bad news for you. The good news is that I've created a lower-sugar version of granola which is just as good (if not better) than the shop-bought alternative. The bad news? It's still just as hard to stop at one serving!

MAKES 10 SERVINGS

300g oats
70g hazelnuts
60g pecans
70g cashews
30g desiccated coconut
2 tbsp coconut oil
60g smooth almond butter
120g honey or agave nectar*
2 tsp cinnamon

Agave nectar is a vegan alternative to honey.

Preheat the oven to 180°C/350°F/gas mark 4.

Combine the oats, nuts and coconut in a bowl.

Mix together the coconut oil, almond butter, honey or agave nectar and cinnamon in another bowl and microwave for 30–45 seconds or until the coconut oil melts. Whisk to combine.

Pour the wet mixture onto the oats and nuts. Stir well.

Spread the mixture out in an even layer on a lined baking tray and press firmly with the back of a spatula. Bake for 15–20 minutes. Remove from the oven, toss the granola with a spatula and place back in the oven to bake for another 10–15 minutes, stirring every few minutes until toasted.

Store in a Kilner jar for up to a week.

PEAR + COCONUT QUINOA PORRIDGE

It's no secret that I love a warm bowl of porridge in the morning, but sometimes I swap my base of oats for quinoa. This grain is high in protein and fibre, which means it helps to keep you full and energised throughout the day.

SERVES 1

50g quinoa, uncooked
125ml water
1 pear
1 tbsp honey, agave nectar or
    sweetener of choice
1 tsp vanilla essence
1 tbsp desiccated coconut, plus
    extra to serve
125ml almond milk*

May be substituted for any milk of your choice.

Rinse the quinoa and place it in a saucepan with the water. Bring to the boil and reduce to simmer for 10 minutes. Cover.

Cut the pear into quarters. Grate ¾ of the pear and slice the last quarter for the top.

Add the grated pear, honey or agave nectar, vanilla essence, coconut and milk to the quinoa and cook for another 5 minutes until thick and creamy.

Pour into a bowl and top with the remaining pear and a sprinkle of coconut.

Serve immediately or store in a box in the fridge to eat cold.

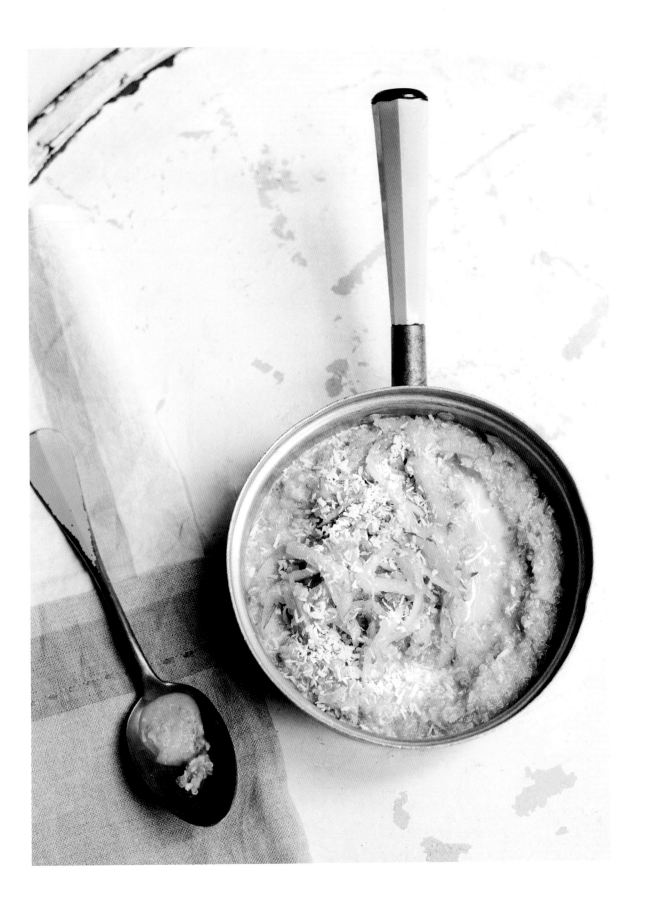

SUPERHERO BIRCHER MUESLI

Why superhero? Because it's brilliantly green and packed full of nutrients. This breakfast will make you feel unstoppable and keep you buzzing until lunchtime. For an extra protein punch, add a tablespoon of protein powder to the mix.

SERVES 1

2 kiwi fruit, peeled and chopped
100ml coconut milk or almond milk
120g natural yogurt (or soya yogurt)
1 tsp matcha powder
1–2 tbsp Stevia, honey or agave nectar
50g oats
Handful of raisins
1 tbsp desiccated coconut

Blend 1 of the kiwis, the coconut or almond milk, yogurt, matcha powder and sweetener in a blender.

In a separate bowl, mix the oats, raisins and coconut.

Stir the kiwi and yogurt mixture into the muesli, add the second kiwi, and pour into a bowl or mason jar.

Allow to set in the fridge overnight or for at least 1–2 hours.

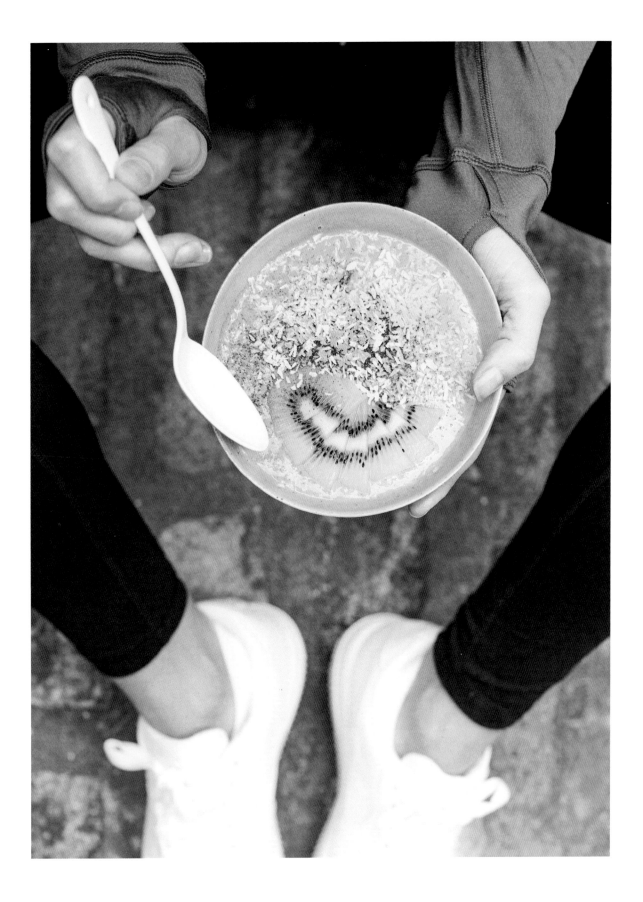

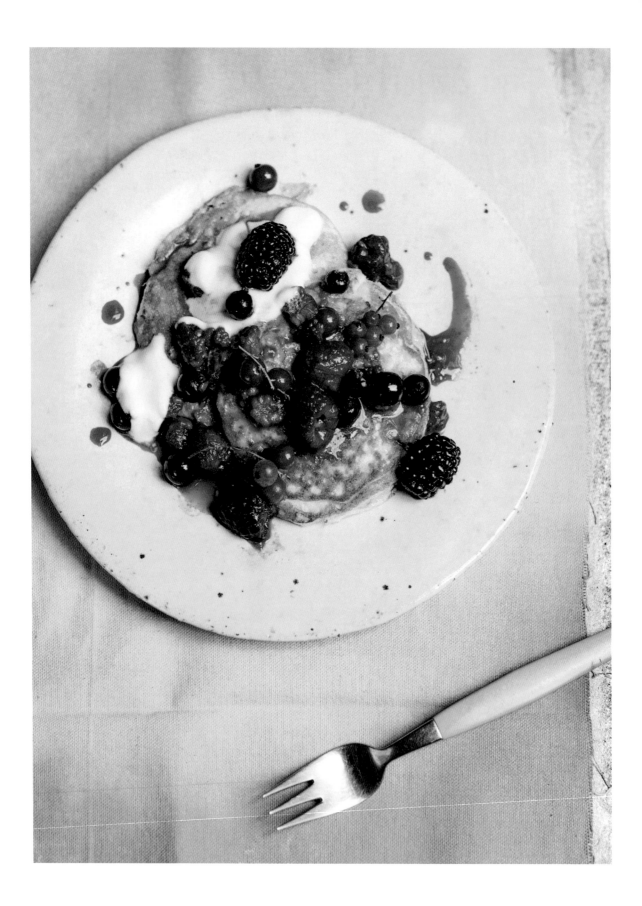

PROTEIN PANCAKES

My favourite Sunday morning breakfast has to be protein pancakes. When I was younger my mum would make us pancakes for breakfast on special occasions like Christmas or our birthdays, so when I have them now as an adult I still feel like it's a treat. However, these pancakes are a lot healthier than the ones we used to have as kids. I like mine best with thick Greek yogurt, warmed berries and lots of cinnamon.

SERVES 2

3 egg whites
60g (2 scoops) protein powder
1 tbsp coconut flour
½ tsp baking powder*
1 banana, mashed
1 tbsp almond milk
1 tbsp coconut oil

Use gluten-free if required.

Whisk the egg whites in a bowl. Mix together all the dry ingredients in a separate bowl, then add the banana and milk, and fold in the egg whites. Stir until there are no clumps and let the mixture sit for 2–3 minutes to thicken.

Melt the coconut oil in a hot non-stick frying pan.

Reduce the heat and add a spoonful of the mixture. Let it cook for 2–4 minutes on each side. Repeat until all the mixture is gone.

ALMOST EMPTY PEANUT BUTTER JAR OVERNIGHT OATS

We've all been there – there's just not enough peanut butter to scrape out of the bottom of the jar with a spoon (or your finger) but there's still too much to warrant throwing the jar away. My solution? Make your oats in the jar, shake it up, and you have instant creamy peanut butter oatmeal – without the washing up!

SERVES 1

50g oats
250ml almond milk
1 tbsp flaxseed or chia seeds
1 tbsp vanilla protein powder*
1 tbsp honey or agave nectar (or sweetener to taste)
1 almost empty jar of peanut butter (or any nut butter!)

Extras: raisins, sliced banana, frozen fruit, cinnamon, nuts or seeds.

* *May be omitted.*

Mix all of the ingredients together in a bowl and pour into the peanut butter jar. Seal with the lid, give it a shake and store in the fridge overnight.

In the morning, add a dash of milk and stir. Top with your favourite extras and eat immediately or after warming up in the microwave.

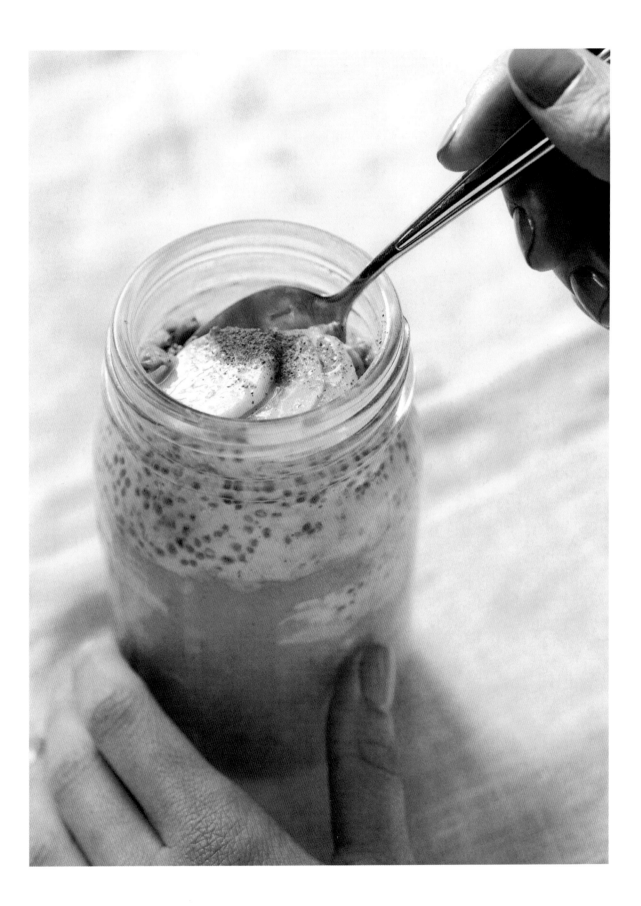

CHOCOLATE + BANANA OVERNIGHT PROTEIN OATS

This is one of my favourite get-up-and-go breakfasts. Prepare it the night before, pop it in the fridge and take it with you to work the next morning. It can be eaten hot or cold and you can play around with the ingredients by adding different fruit, nuts, seeds or flavoured protein powders.

SERVES 2

1 banana, mashed
100g oats
300ml unsweetened vanilla
    almond milk
25g chocolate protein powder*
1 tbsp unsweetened cocoa powder
1 tbsp chia seeds
2 squares of 85 per cent dark
    chocolate, grated
a few slices of banana, to serve

* May be omitted.

Put the mashed banana, oats, almond milk, protein powder, cocoa powder and chia seeds into a bowl. Stir well and pour the mixture into 2 containers with lids (jam jars work well). Store overnight in the fridge.

Take the jars out of the fridge and give them a stir. Add more almond milk if the mixture appears too thick. Sprinkle over the dark chocolate and place a few extra slices of banana on top.

Grab your spoons and go!

SCRAMBLED EGGS + SMOKED SALMON IN PORTOBELLO MUSHROOM BOATS

How do you like your eggs in the morning? I like mine every way! These mushroom boats are perfect not only for holding scrambled eggs but poached, baked or fried eggs too. The mushroom base makes the perfect light alternative to traditional eggs on toast or crumpets.

SERVES 1

2 Portobello mushrooms
1 tbsp extra-virgin olive oil
2 free-range eggs
1 tbsp almond milk
1 tbsp chives, chopped
¼ tsp salt
¼ tsp black pepper
½ tbsp butter or coconut oil
50g smoked salmon, sliced into ribbons
1 spring onion, finely chopped, to serve

Preheat the oven to 180°C/350°F/gas mark 4.

Brush the mushrooms with olive oil. Place them face up on a baking sheet and roast for 15 minutes. Pour out any liquid that has accumulated in the caps. Set aside.

Whisk the eggs, milk, chives, salt and pepper together.

Put a small pan over a low heat and melt the butter or coconut oil.

Pour the beaten eggs into the pan. Stir slowly using a spatula, bringing in all the mixture from the edges of the pan. Continue to stir until the eggs are cooked. Stir in the smoked salmon.

Divide the scrambled eggs and salmon between the mushrooms. Sprinkle the spring onion over the filled mushroom boats and serve.

CHOPPED EGG + AVO SALAD ON RYE TOAST

When we had guests arrive at our door without warning, my mum would usher us into the kitchen to help her make up a batch of chopped egg salad sandwiches. I loved this recipe as child and I still do as an adult, but I've made a few tweaks to the recipe to give it a healthy 'Food Medic' twist. The beauty of this chopped salad is that the ingredients are usually in your fridge already so it doesn't require running out to the shops when you're rushing around in the morning. I often make it the night before and then pile it on top of my rye toast in the morning. This also works great inside a wrap for lunch.

SERVES 1

2 boiled eggs, cooled and chopped
½ avocado, diced
1 salad tomato, diced
1 spring onion, finely chopped
1 tbsp natural yogurt
Salt and black pepper, to taste

TO SERVE
1 slice of rye bread (or bread of choice)

Put all the ingredients into a mixing bowl and mash roughly with a fork.

Toast the bread and spoon the egg salad on top.

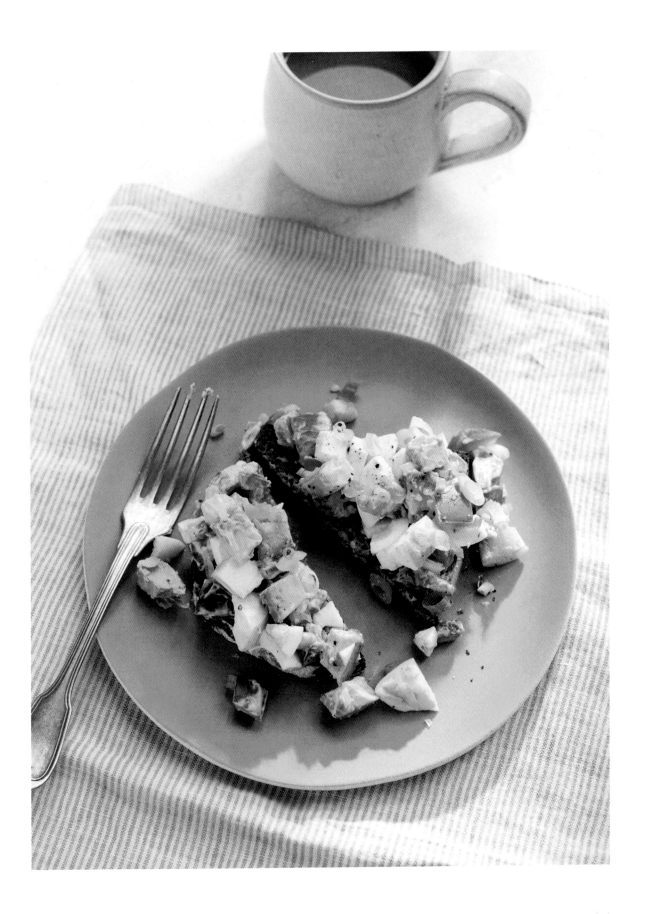

SWEET POTATO + CHORIZO HASH WITH BAKED EGGS

When I have a little more time on the weekends to make a lazy breakfast, this is one of my favourite dishes. The oil from the chorizo really adds an incredible Spanish flavour to the dish but for a veggie alternative, sundried tomatoes also do the trick.

SERVES 2

1 tbsp coconut oil
½ red onion, diced
1 small sweet potato (200–300g), chopped into small cubes.
50g chorizo, diced
Handful of kale
2 free-range eggs
Salt and black pepper

Preheat the oven to 180°C/350°F/gas mark 4.

Heat the coconut oil in a large frying pan. Add the red onion and sweet potato. Fry over a medium heat for 10 minutes or until the sweet potato is cooked.

Add the chorizo and kale, and cook for another 5 minutes. Season with salt and pepper.

Transfer the sweet potato mixture to an ovenproof dish and crack the eggs on top. Bake in the oven for 10–12 minutes or until the eggs are cooked.

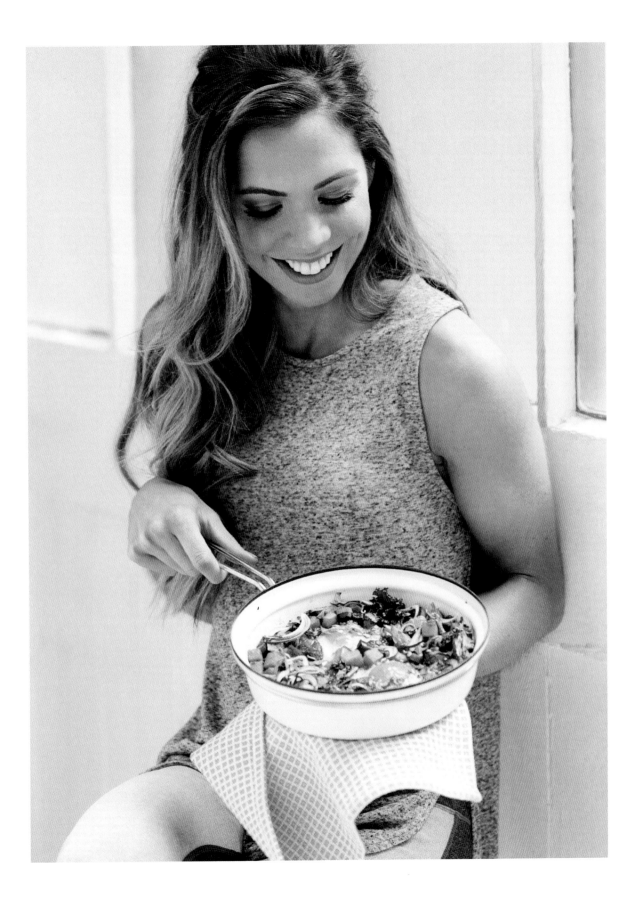

AMERICAN-STYLE PANCAKES WITH BACON AND SYRUP

This recipe makes the fluffiest, healthiest pancakes that you will ever have! These pancakes sound seriously indulgent but are wonderfully light, low in carbohydrates and naturally gluten-free. If you're not a fan of the sweet and salty combo of bacon and syrup, they are also tasty served with sweet sides, such as blueberries, banana and yogurt.

SERVES 1

3 tbsp coconut flour
1 tbsp coconut sugar or sweetener of choice
¼ tsp baking powder*
3 egg whites
1 tsp vanilla extract
1 tbsp apple sauce
100–120ml almond milk
1 tbsp coconut oil
Salt

TO SERVE
2 smoked or maple-cured rashers of bacon
Toasted pecans, to sprinkle
Maple syrup or honey, to drizzle

Use gluten-free if required.

In a large bowl, combine the coconut flour, sugar or sweetener, baking powder and a pinch of salt.

In a separate mixing bowl, whisk the egg whites for 2–3 minutes. The longer you whisk, the fluffier the pancake.

Add the egg whites to the dry mixture along with the vanilla extract and apple sauce. Fold together. The batter will form a paste-like texture.

Next add the milk, 1 tablespoon at a time to achieve the desired consistency (be patient as this may take a few minutes).

Add the coconut oil to a greaseproof pan and place over a medium–low heat. Spoon the batter into the pan, 2 tablespoons at a time. You should have enough batter to make 4–5 small pancakes. The batter is quite delicate, so smaller pancakes will be easier to turn.

Cook the pancakes for 2–3 minutes on 1 side before flipping, and cooking on the other side for another 2 minutes or until the pancakes are golden. If you find that the pancakes are beginning to brown too quickly, reduce the heat.

Serve with the bacon, a scattering of pecans and a drizzle of syrup or honey.

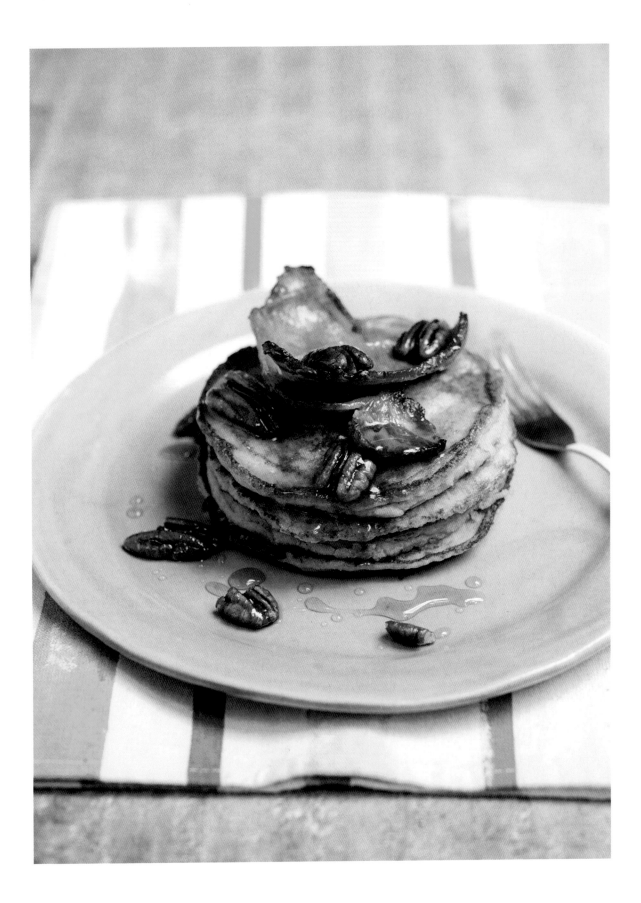

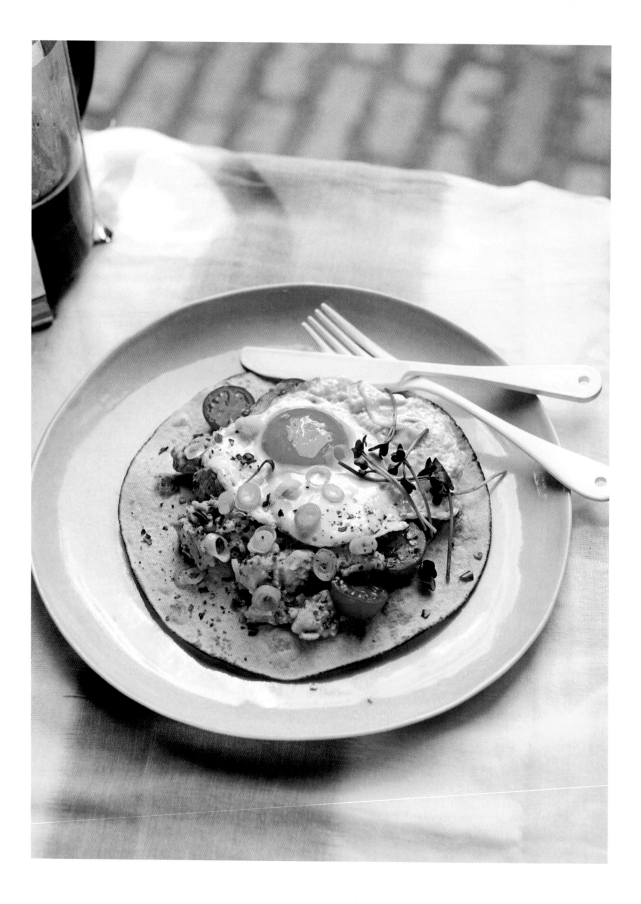

MEXICAN BREAKFAST WRAP

This recipe was created unintentionally one day when I had minimal ingredients in the fridge and had to be creative. The result was absolutely delicious and, incidentally, super-healthy, so I've been making it on a regular basis ever since.

SERVES 1

½ ripe avocado, chopped
¼ tsp chilli flakes
1 tbsp lemon juice (approx ½ lemon)
1 garlic clove, finely chopped
1 tbsp coconut oil
1 free-range egg
1 corn tortilla
4 cherry tomatoes, halved
½ spring onion, finely chopped
Salt and black pepper

Place the avocado, chilli flakes, lemon juice and garlic in a small bowl and mash with a fork. Add a pinch of salt and black pepper to taste.

Heat the coconut oil in a frying pan and crack the egg into the pan. Fry for 5 minutes until cooked.

Place the wrap under a hot grill and lightly toast for 2–3 minutes.

Spoon the smashed avocado into the centre of the wrap to create a small circle. Put the tomatoes onto the avocado and place the egg on top. Sprinkle with the spring onion and serve.

GOAT'S CHEESE + MINTED GREENS FRITTATA

This recipe is good for breakfast, brunch, lunch or dinner. I like to make it in advance and pop it in a lunchbox to take to work with me. If goat's cheese isn't your cup of tea, cheeses like feta and mozzarella also work well. Don't be afraid to add in any extra veggies that are sitting in the fridge.

SERVES 4

150g frozen peas
8 free-range eggs
75ml almond milk
1 large courgette (approx 200g), grated
Handful of fresh mint, roughly chopped
1 tbsp coconut oil
80g goat's cheese
Salt and black pepper

Preheat the oven to 200°C/400°F/gas mark 6.

Boil the peas for 5 minutes in a saucepan of water. Drain and set aside.

In a large bowl, whisk the eggs and the milk together. Stir in the courgette, peas and mint, and season with salt and pepper.

Place a large ovenproof frying pan over a medium heat and add the coconut oil. Pour in the egg mix and gently cook for 8–10 minutes until the base and sides are cooked.

Slice the goat's cheese into 4 even circles and place on the top of the frittata. Crumble any remaining goat's cheese on top.

Place the pan in the oven for 10–15 minutes until the top is golden and the cheese is bubbling.

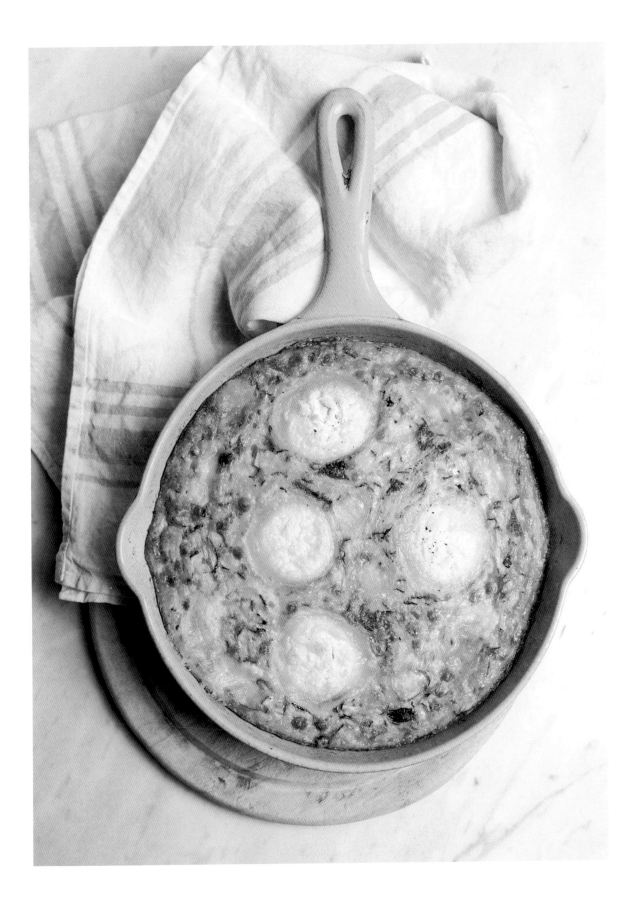

SHAKES
+
SMOOTHIES

There are no rules when it comes to a smoothie.

Shakes and smoothies are a great way to get in a balanced meal full of vitamins, minerals, fibre, lean protein and healthy fats, and really, anything goes – so don't be afraid to experiment. In the same way that I showed you how to create a balanced plate, I've come up with a special formula to help you build the perfect smoothie. If you're in need of a little inspiration, I've included ten of my favourite smoothie and shake recipes. All the recipes serve 1.

STEP 1

Pick your base: water, coconut water, almond milk

STEP 2

Choose 2–3 portions of fruit and vegetables

STEP 3

Add a protein: whey protein, vegan protein, Greek yogurt, Quark or cottage cheese

STEP 4

Accessorise with fat: a tablespoon of peanut butter or almond butter, half an avocado, a tablespoon of flax or chia seeds, a handful of nuts

TIP: *Use frozen fruit and veg for a thicker smoothie.*

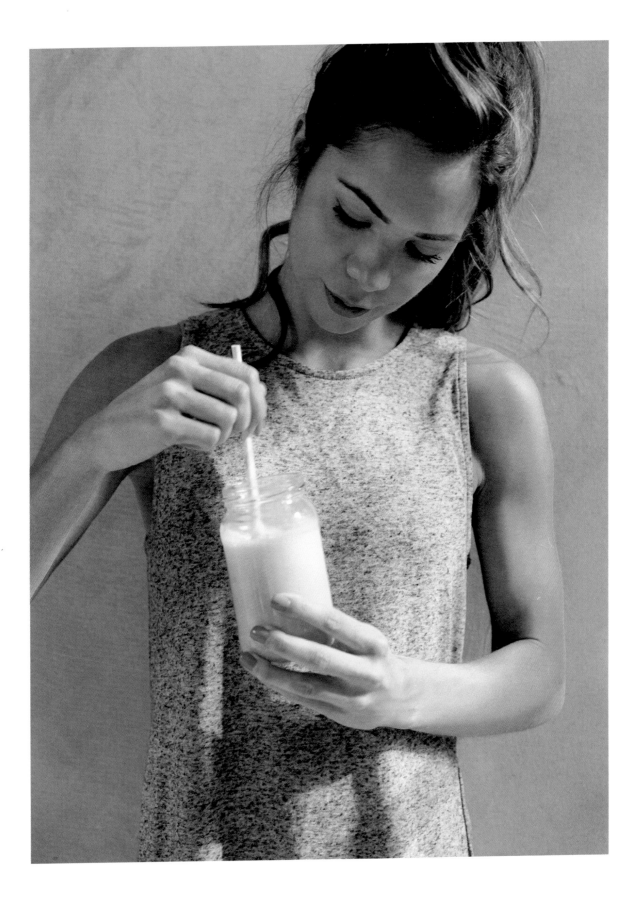

HIGH-PROTEIN PIÑA COLADA

1 banana, frozen
100g fresh pineapple
200ml coconut water
25g (1 scoop) vanilla protein
   powder
1 heaped tbsp desiccated coconut

Place all the ingredients together
in a blender and combine until
well mixed.

BANOFFEE PIE SMOOTHIE

½ tsp cinnamon
1 banana, frozen
1 tbsp honey or agave nectar
30g pecan nuts
200ml unsweetened almond milk

Place all the ingredients together
in a blender and combine until
well mixed.

PEANUT BUTTERCUP PROTEIN SHAKE

25g (1 scoop) vanilla protein
   powder
200ml unsweetened almond milk
1 frozen banana
2 tbsp peanut flour*
2 tbsp cocoa powder
Handful of ice cubes

Place all the ingredients together
in a blender and combine until
well mixed.

*May be substituted for 1 tbsp of
peanut butter.

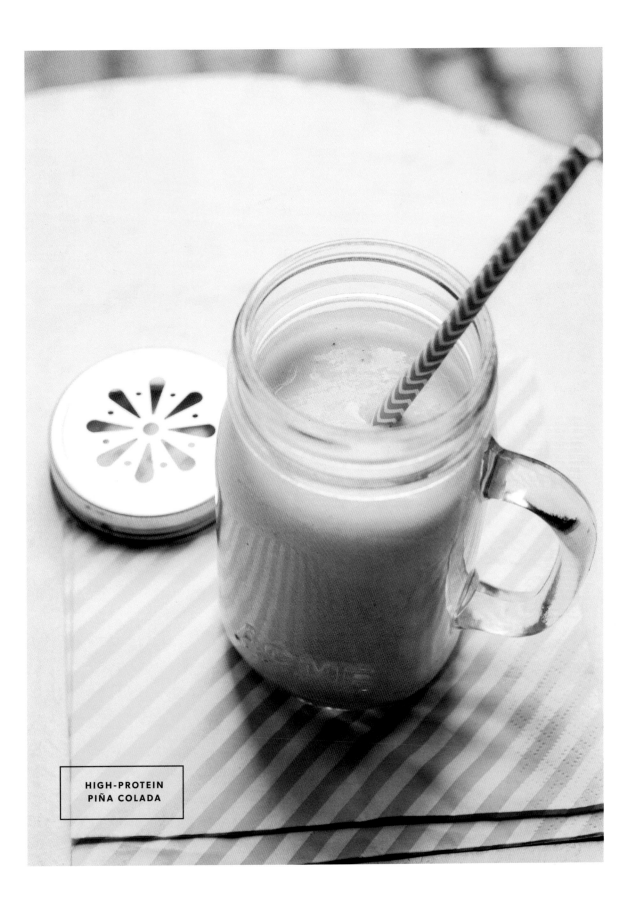

HIGH-PROTEIN
PIÑA COLADA

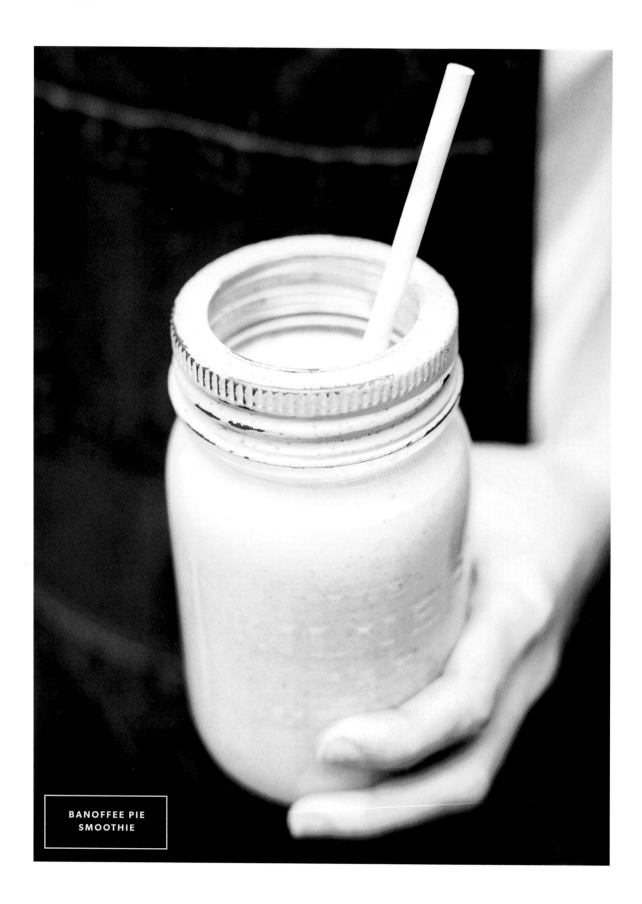

BANOFFEE PIE
SMOOTHIE

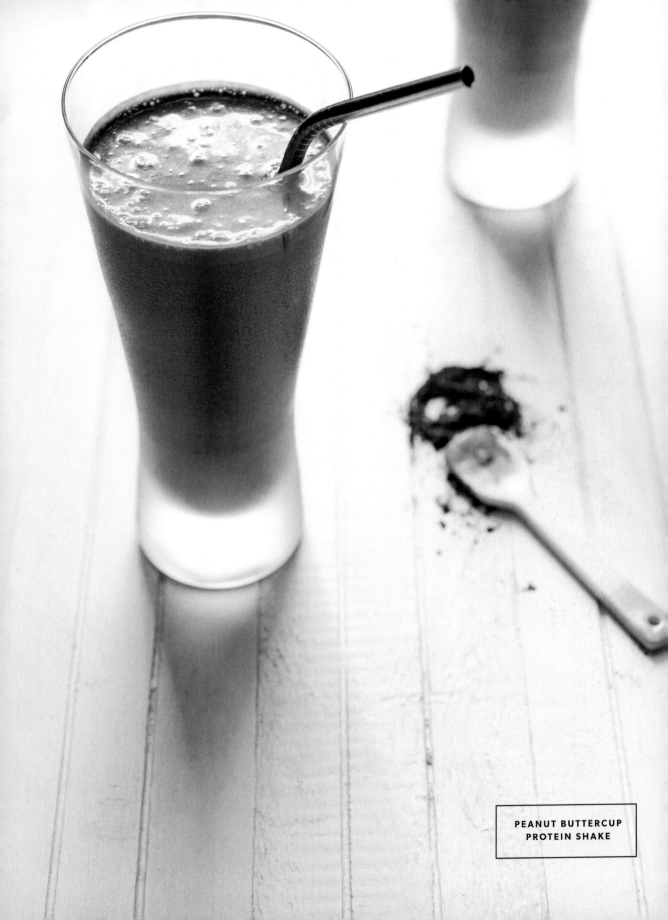

PEANUT BUTTERCUP
PROTEIN SHAKE

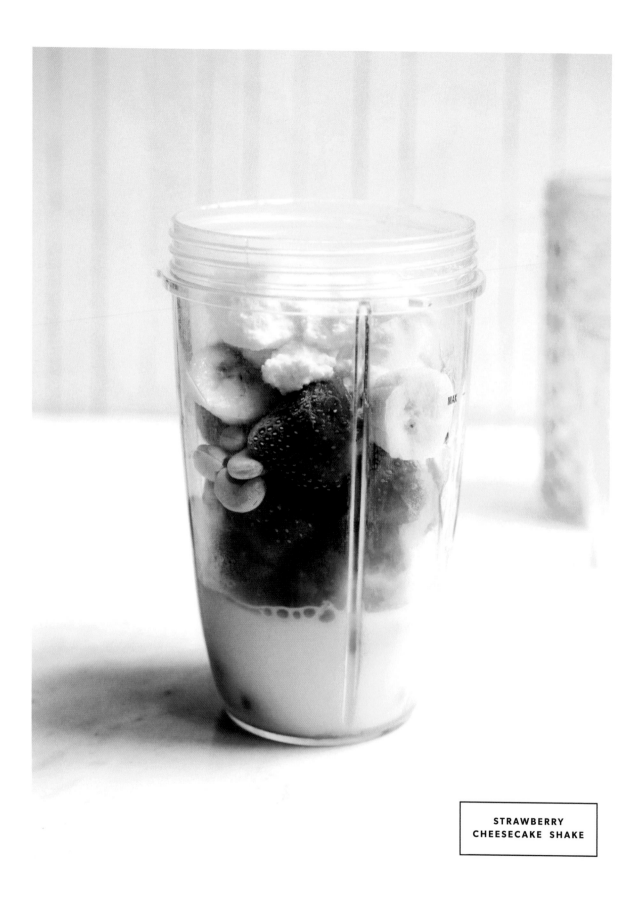

STRAWBERRY
CHEESECAKE SHAKE

STRAWBERRY CHEESECAKE SHAKE

30g cashews
100g frozen strawberries (or raspberries)
200ml unsweetened almond milk
100g Quark or Greek yogurt
½ frozen banana
1 tbsp honey or agave nectar
Handful of ice cubes

Place the cashews in a blender and pulse until finely chopped.

Add the rest of the ingredients to the blender and combine until well mixed.

THE HULK SHAKE

25g (1 scoop) vanilla protein powder
1 ripe banana, chopped
2 handfuls of fresh curly kale
1 tbsp almond butter or peanut butter
250ml unsweetened almond milk
Handful of ice cubes

Place all the ingredients together in a blender and combine until well mixed.

PINK BEET + BERRY SHAKE

1 frozen banana
100g frozen strawberries (or raspberries)
1 large cooked beetroot
200ml unsweetened almond milk

Place all the ingredients together in a blender and combine until well mixed.

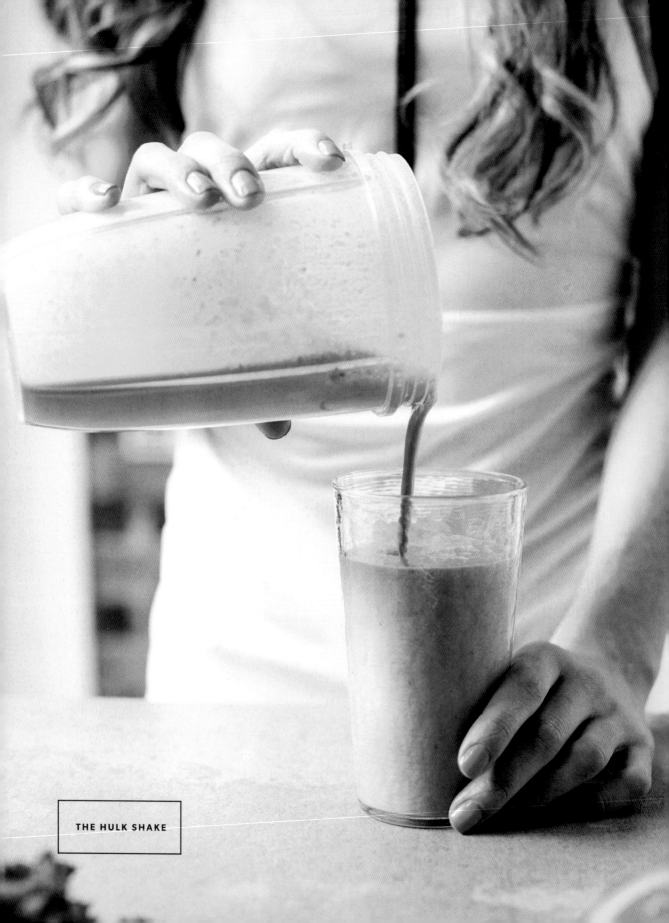

THE HULK SHAKE

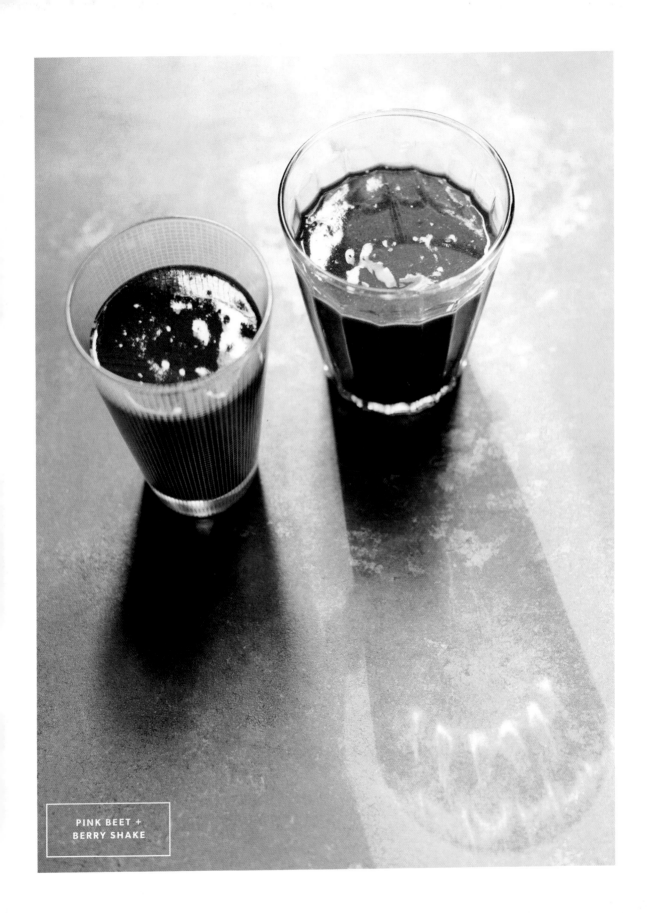

PINK BEET +
BERRY SHAKE

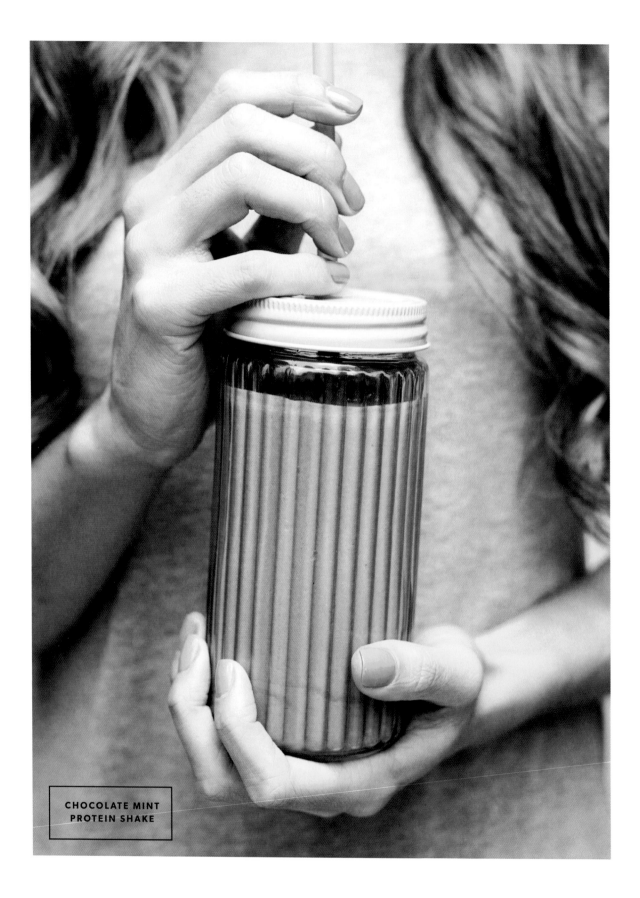

CHOCOLATE MINT
PROTEIN SHAKE

CHOCOLATE MINT PROTEIN SHAKE

½ medium avocado, chopped
25g (1 scoop) chocolate protein
 powder
2 tbsp cocoa powder
300ml unsweetened almond milk
½ tsp peppermint extract
Handful of ice cubes
Mint leaves, to garnish (*optional*)

Place all the ingredients together
in a blender and combine until
well mixed.

MANGO MATCHA MUSCLE MAKER

25g (1 scoop) vanilla protein
 powder
100g frozen mango
60g frozen spinach*
1 ripe banana, chopped
½ tsp matcha powder
200ml unsweetened almond milk

Place all the ingredients together
in a blender and combine until
well mixed.

** May be swapped for 2 handfuls
of fresh spinach and a handful of
ice cubes.*

BLUEBERRY MUFFIN PROTEIN SHAKE

80g frozen blueberries
20g oats
1 tbsp peanut butter
2 dates, chopped
25g (1 scoop) vanilla protein
 powder
200ml unsweetened almond milk
½ tsp cinnamon
Handful of ice cubes

Place all the ingredients together
in a blender and combine until
well mixed.

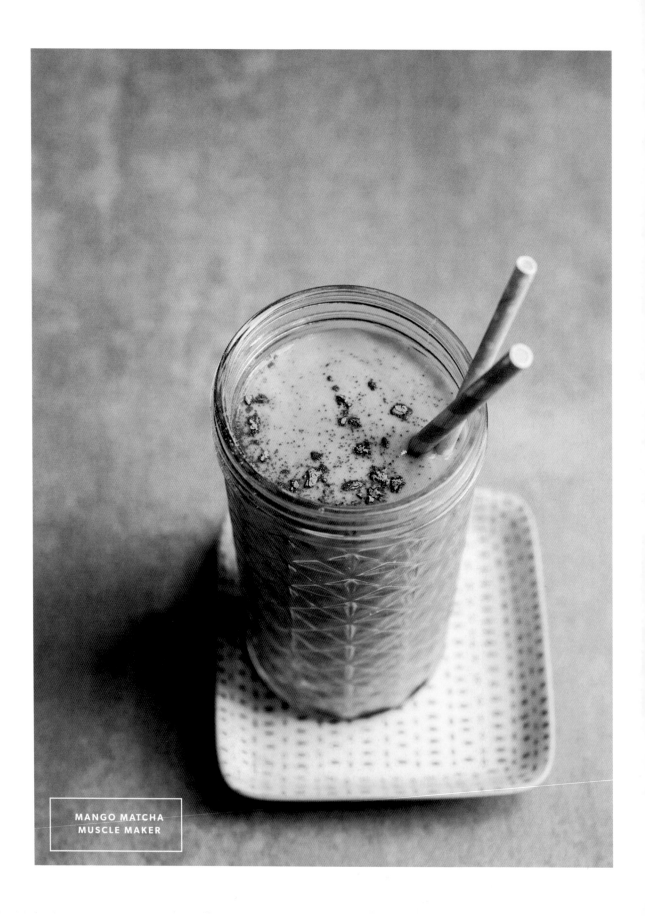

MANGO MATCHA
MUSCLE MAKER

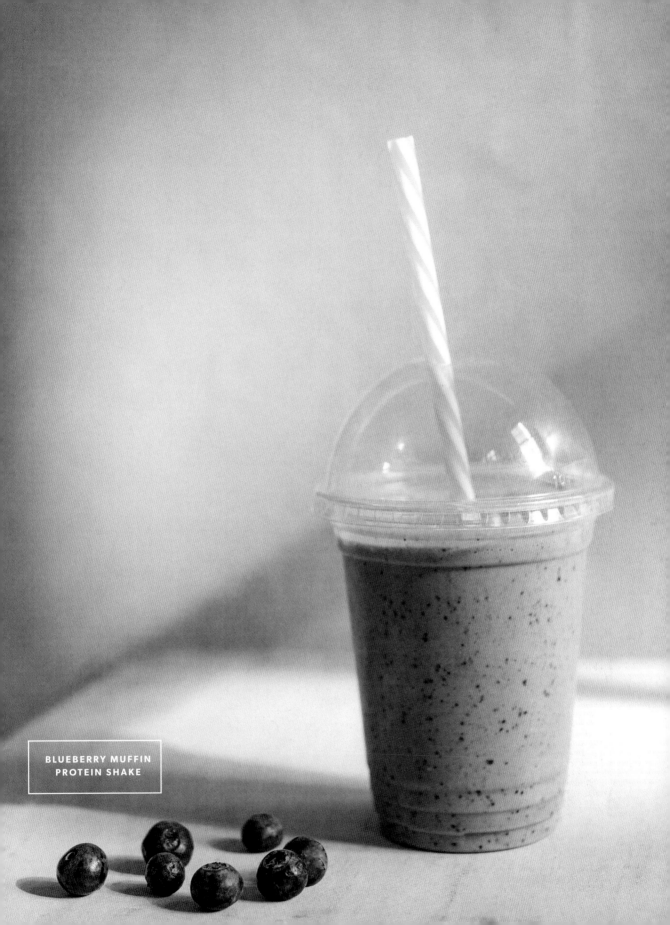

BLUEBERRY MUFFIN
PROTEIN SHAKE

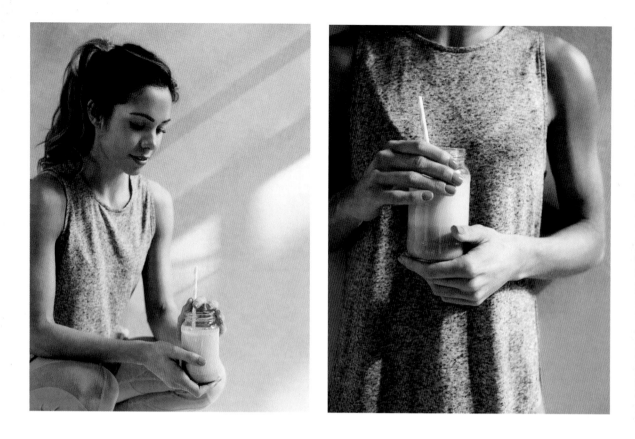

ICED PROTEIN COFFEE

25g (1 scoop) vanilla protein powder
1 shot of brewed strong coffee, chilled
250ml unsweetened almond milk
Handful of ice cubes
2–3 caramel or vanilla Stevia flavoured
    drops (*optional*)

Place all the ingredients together in a blender and combine until
well mixed.

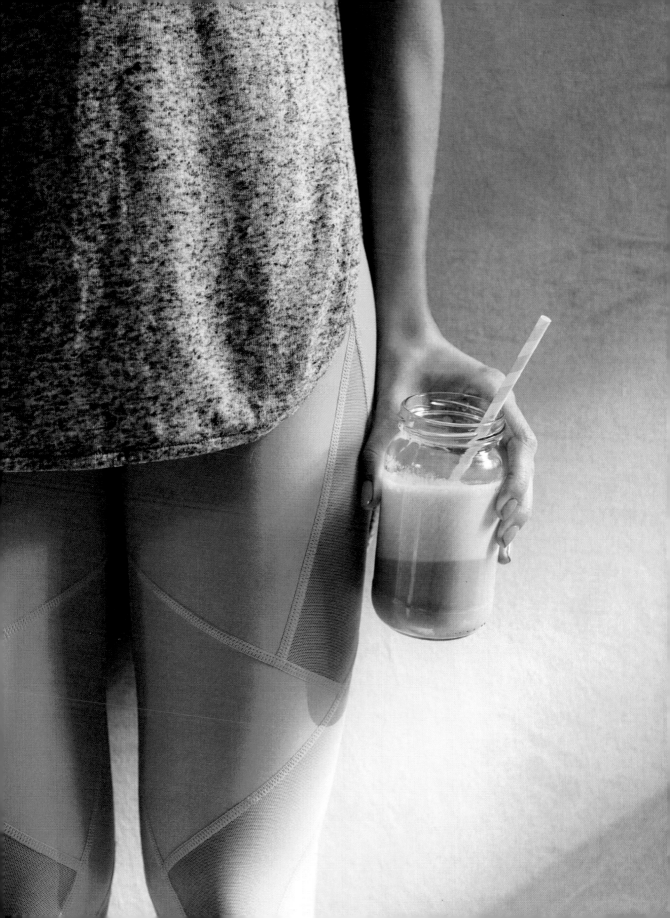

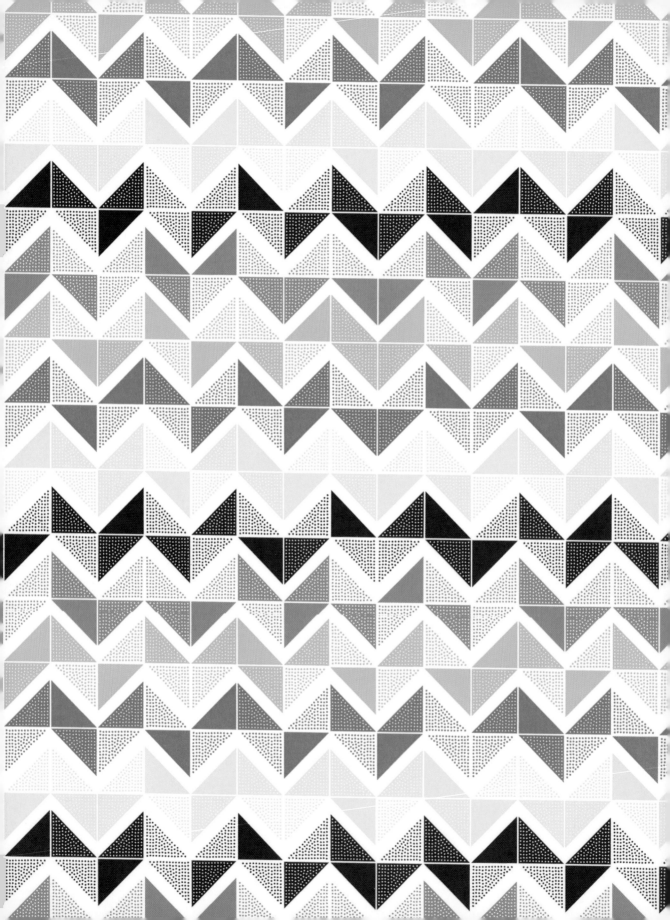

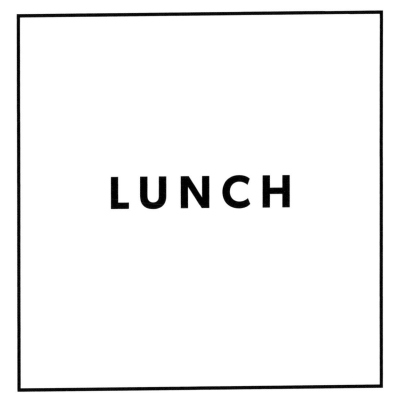

LUNCH

I'm always that girl who brings a packed lunch with me!

I would much rather make my own salad for lunch than spend a fortune on a shop-bought, limp salad, made up of a few lettuce leaves, a slice or two of chicken and buckets of sugary dressing.

My lunches tend to be lighter than my dinners so you may notice that they are lower in starchy carbohydrates than the dinner recipes in this book. I personally find that having a lighter lunch, packed full of wholesome food, boosts my energy whilst helping me to avoid that post-lunch 3 p.m. slump.

But don't worry – these lunches are not going to leave you hungry! They are designed to leave you totally satisfied, and will have you counting down the hours until lunchtime. Packed full of protein, fresh vegetables and heart-healthy fats, you'll never want to buy another 'meal-deal' for lunch again. From teriyaki beef and Asian-style broccoli rice (page 146) to summery puy lentil, feta and mint salad (page 163), there's lots to choose from, whatever mood you're in and whatever dietary preference you have.

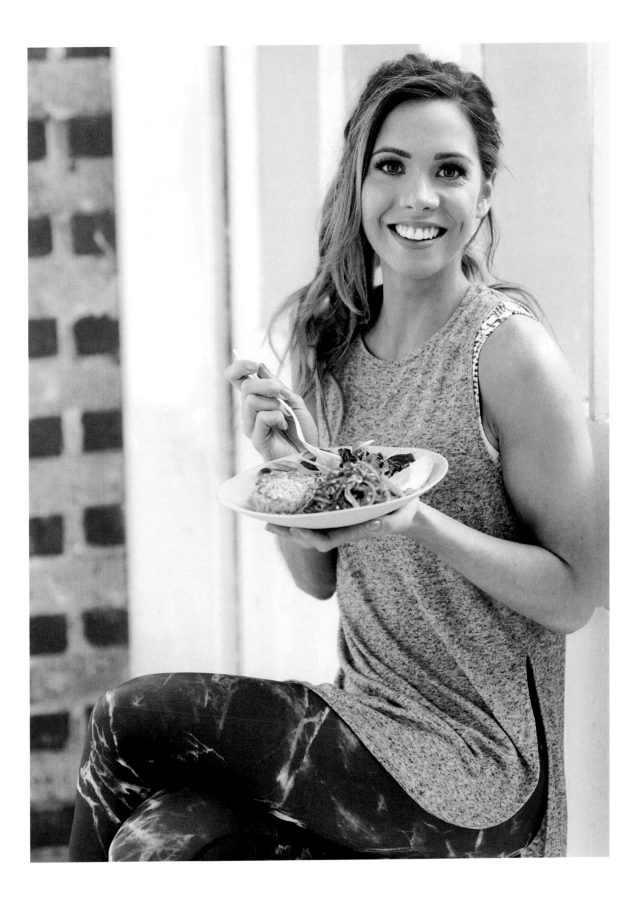

TANDOORI CHICKPEA + COURGETTE BURGERS

It's no secret that I'm a big meat eater, but there's something about a veggie burger that is just so satisfying and moreish that I find myself craving this over a beef burger.

The base of this burger is chickpeas, a staple ingredient in my cupboard and in many of my recipes. They're packed full of protein, so make a great meat alternative, not to mention all the fibre, vitamins, and minerals they contain. This recipe also works well as a brunch option with a runny poached egg served on top.

MAKES 5–6 BURGERS

1 small onion, diced
1 garlic clove, crushed or grated
2 tbsp coconut oil
1 x 400g tin of chickpeas, rinsed
  and drained
½ courgette, grated
1 tbsp tahini
1–2 tbsp Oatly milk
50g oats
½ tsp turmeric
½ tsp ground cumin
½ tsp chilli powder
Salt and black pepper

TO SERVE
Salad of your choice

Fry the onion and garlic in a teaspoon of the coconut oil until soft and translucent.

Place the chickpeas in a food processor along with the courgette, tahini, milk, oats and seasoning, to taste. Pulse until they are combined, but not completely smooth, to retain a bit of texture.

Divide the mixture into 5 or 6 palm-sized burgers. Place on a tray in the fridge for 30–60 minutes to firm up. Preheat the oven to 180°C/350°F/gas mark 4.

Heat the remaining coconut oil in a non-stick frying pan and cook the burgers for about 5–10 minutes on both sides to crisp up the outside and seal in the moisture.

Place the burgers on a tray lined with greaseproof paper and bake in the oven for 20–25 minutes.

Serve these up with a salad of your choice. I love mine alongside lettuce, tomatoes, alfafa sprouts and avocado.

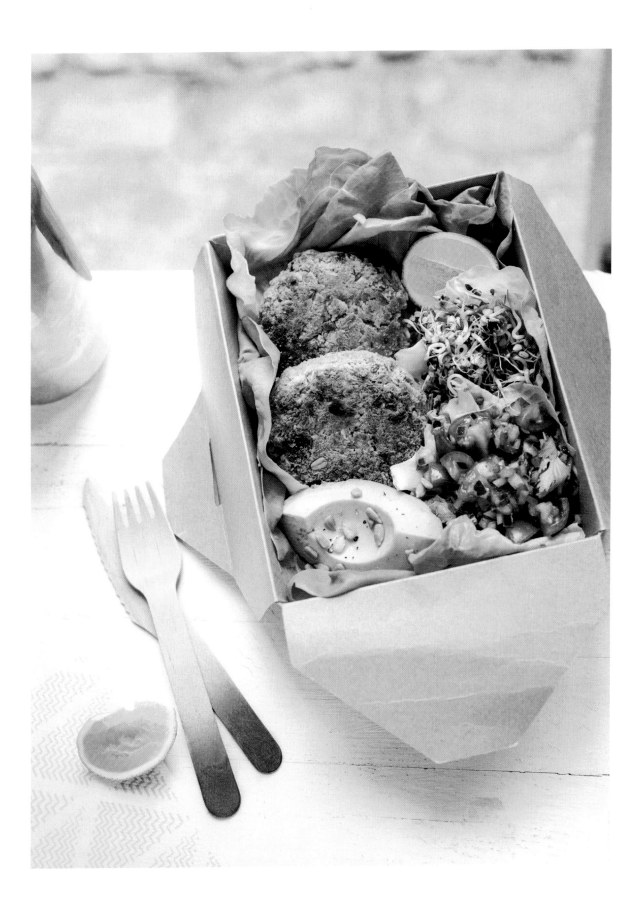

FETA, AUBERGINE, POMEGRANATE + HARISSA SALAD

This Moroccan-inspired salad is really delicious with a combination of different flavours from the juicy roasted aubergines, creamy feta and sweet pomegranate seeds.

Aubergines are one of my favourite vegetables – but only when they're cooked right. In my opinion, the best way to have them is grilled or roasted. Aubergine is perfect for grilling on the barbecue or roasting in the oven due to their squishy texture, which acts like a sponge, soaking up all the oils and seasoning.

SERVES 2

1 aubergine
½ white onion, diced
1 garlic clove, crushed
1–2 tbsp extra-virgin olive oil
1 bunch of cavolo nero or kale
100g quinoa, cooked
Juice of ½ lemon
1 tsp tahini
1 tsp harissa paste
80g pomegranate seeds
100g feta cheese
Salt and black pepper

Preheat the oven to 180°C/350°F/gas mark 4.

Slice the aubergine lengthways into approximately 16 strips. Brush with a little of the olive oil and sprinkle with salt and pepper. Roast for 30 minutes, tossing midway to cook both sides.

Fry the onion and garlic over a low heat with a tablespoon of olive oil.

Cut the cavolo nero leaves free from the core and slice out any tough central stalks. Add the leaves and cooked aubergine to the pan with the onion and garlic, and sauté over a low heat for 2–3 minutes. Add the quinoa and cook for a further 5 minutes.

Transfer the salad to a large bowl.

Whisk the lemon juice, tahini and harissa paste in a separate bowl and drizzle on top of the warm salad. Mix well.

Sprinkle over the pomegranate seeds and crumbled feta cheese, and serve immediately, or alternatively, store in the fridge and eat cold later.

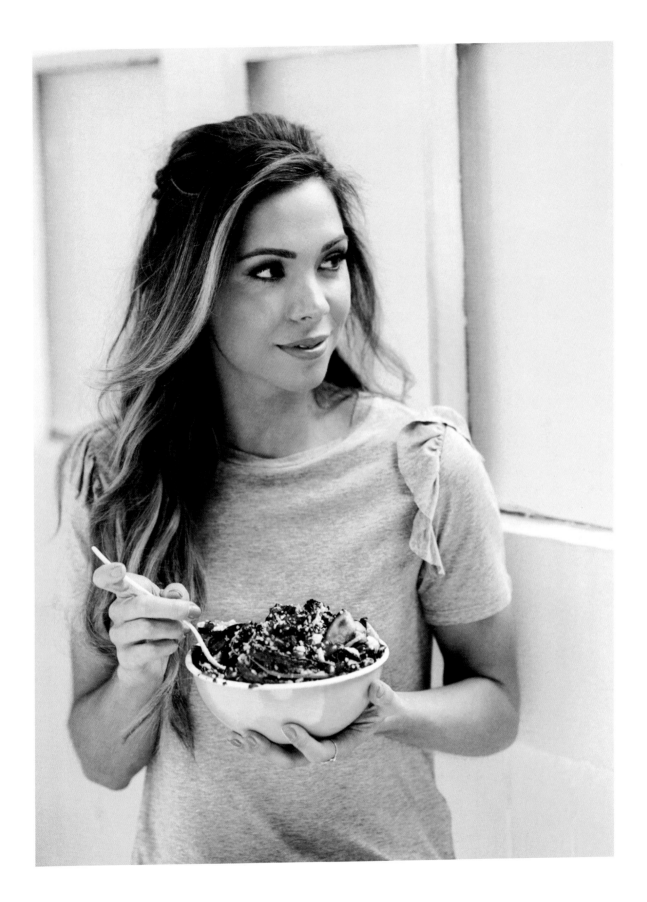

ZESTY CARROT + ORANGE SOUP

There's nothing more comforting than a big bowl of soup and some freshly baked bread to dunk into it. This soup is very light and summery, so you don't have to wait for the winter months to try it out. I serve it with some crumbled feta cheese and a thick slice of my rosemary seeded bread (see page 139).

SERVES 6

2 tbsp coconut oil
1 large white onion, diced
1 celery stalk, diced
1 garlic clove, grated
8 carrots, peeled and chopped
Juice and zest of 1 orange
1 litre vegetable stock
50ml almond milk
Salt and black pepper

Place a large saucepan over a medium heat and add the coconut oil. Cook the onion, celery and garlic until soft.

Add the carrots, season with salt and pepper, and add the orange zest.

Add the stock and bring to the boil. Cover and allow to simmer for 30–35 minutes until the carrots are soft.

Using a hand blender, blend the mixture until smooth, or ladle carefully into a food processor and blend until smooth. Now add the juice of the orange and the milk.

Season with salt and pepper to taste.

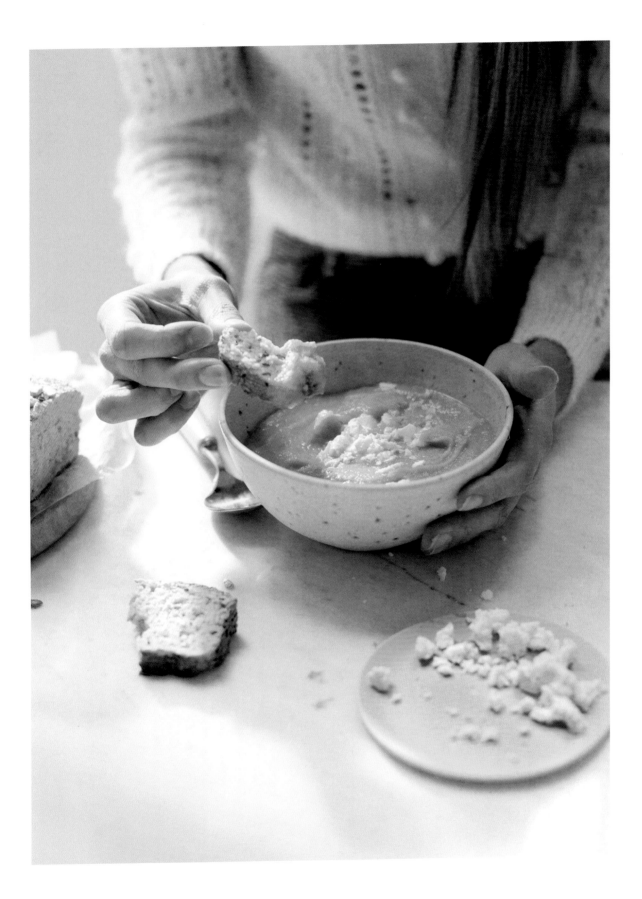

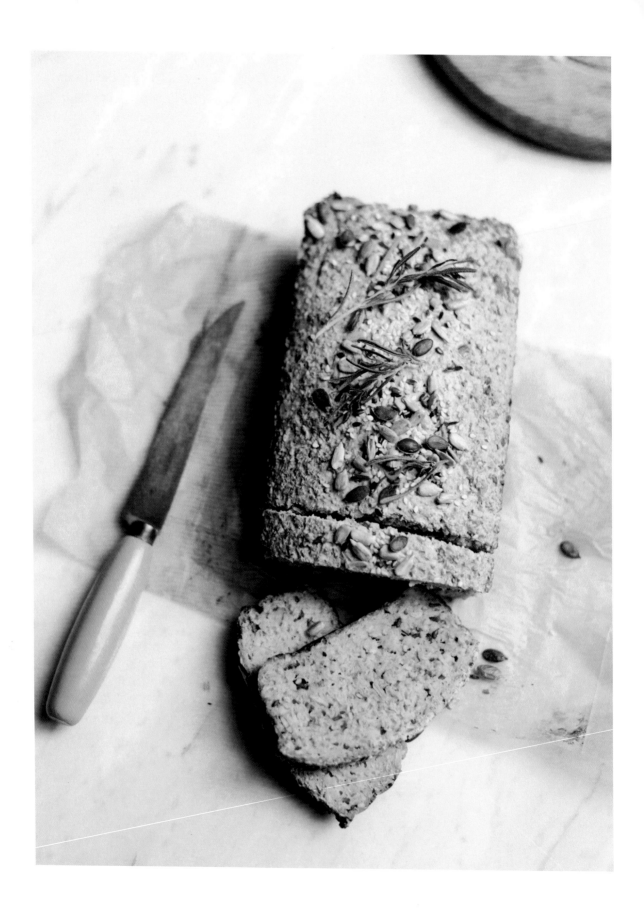

ROSEMARY + MIXED SEED BREAD

There's nothing quite like freshly baked bread and for lots of people, shop-bought bread isn't always the easiest thing to digest. This recipe is low in sugar and made with only a handful of ingredients, which you can find in any supermarket. I like to season mine with rosemary but basil works wonderfully too. Serve it with some home-made soup for lunch (see page 136) or with some poached eggs for breakfast.

MAKES 8–10 SLICES

300g oats
80g mixed seeds
1 tsp baking powder*
1 tsp pink Himalayan salt
500g natural yogurt
1 free-range egg
1 tsp coconut oil, melted
1 tbsp finely chopped rosemary

Use gluten-free if required.

Preheat the oven to 180°C/350°F/gas mark 4.

Combine the dry ingredients in a bowl and then stir in the yogurt and egg.

Grease a bread tin or silicone tray with the coconut oil (silicone trays work best).

Pour the mixture in and bake for 30 minutes. Turn the oven temperature down to 150°C/300°F/gas mark 2 and bake for a further 20–25 minutes.

PEANUT BUTTER HUMMUS

(centred)

The addition of creamy peanut butter takes your regular hummus to a whole new level! I don't think enough people make their own hummus – often they don't realise how easy it is to make. I store it in a tub in the fridge to snack on with raw carrots and peppers.

SERVES 4 ─────────────────

1 x 400g tin of chickpeas, rinsed
   and drained
Juice of 1 lemon
2 tbsp crunchy peanut butter
1 tbsp tahini
1 tbsp extra-virgin olive oil
2 garlic cloves
½ tsp smoked paprika
½ tsp salt
80ml unsweetened almond milk
1 tbsp mixed seeds, to garnish
   (optional)

Place all the ingredients into a food processor and blend until creamy. Garnish with a sprinkle of mixed seeds.

PS... The peanut butter can be swapped for cashew nut butter.

CREAMY AUBERGINE DIP

(top right)

This is my simple, healthier version of the classic Middle Eastern dish baba ganoush. I love drizzling this on top of roasted cauliflower, or using it as a spread on rye bread with chicken, or simply for dipping my veggies into.

MAKES 4 SERVINGS ─────────────────

1 whole aubergine
2 garlic cloves, crushed or grated
¼ tsp smoked paprika, plus a little
   extra to garnish
2 heaped tbsp Greek yogurt
1 tbsp tahini
Juice of ½ lemon
½ –1 tsp salt (or to taste)

Preheat the oven to 200°C/400°F/gas mark 6.

Place the aubergine on a flat baking tray. Roast for 45 minutes, turning halfway through. Remove from the oven and allow to cool for an hour.

Once cool, peel the skin from the aubergine and place the flesh in a food processor or blender. Add the rest of the ingredients to the blend and combine until smooth.

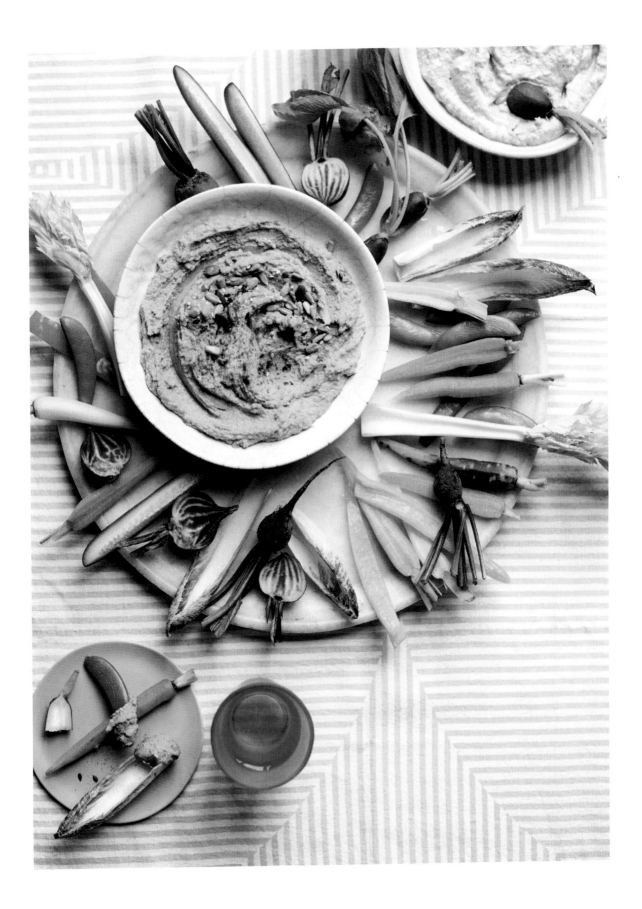

MEXICAN CHICKEN SALAD BOWL

I actually made this salad on a whim – it was a spur-of-the-moment, what-do-I-have-in-my-fridge kind of thing! I often think that those are the recipes that sometimes work out the best. I had some roast chicken in the fridge, and a tin of kidney beans in the cupboard so something Mexican came to mind.

Mexican food is hands-down my favourite cuisine – beans, cheese, guacamole, peppers and of course, nachos! Unfortunately, my body would not thank me for eating nachos on a regular basis so this is where I need to be creative so that I can keep my healthy diet on track, and still satisfy my cravings.

SERVES 2

FOR THE DRESSING
Juice of 1 lime
2 tbsp olive oil
¼ tsp smoked paprika
½ tsp chilli powder
¼ tsp black pepper
Salt

FOR THE SALAD
½ 240g tin of kidney beans, drained and rinsed
1 x 160g tin of sweetcorn, drained
1 small red onion, diced
1 salad tomato, chopped
1 red pepper, chopped
¼ 200g jar of jalapeños in brine, drained
½ iceberg lettuce head, shredded
2 grilled boneless, skinless chicken breasts, sliced
1 ripe avocado, sliced

First, make the dressing by whisking together the ingredients in a small bowl.

Place the kidney beans, sweetcorn, red onion, tomato, red pepper and jalapeños in a large mixing bowl. Pour the dressing over the ingredients and mix well.

Separate the lettuce into 2 serving bowls, add half the chopped salad to each bowl, and top each salad with the chicken and avocado slices.

PS... This salad works great layered in a Kilner jar. Add the dressing first, followed by the salad, avocado and finally the chicken on top.

SALMON + ASPARAGUS SALAD NIÇOISE

This salad is so fresh and so light, but oh-so-satisfying. I feel like a total goddess after I eat it with all those healthy fats from the salmon, eggs and olives. It's not heavy on starchy carbohydrates or fibre, which makes it very gentle on the gut.

SERVES 1

FOR THE SALAD
2 fresh salmon fillets
300g baby potatoes (about 8)
100g asparagus tips
2 free-range eggs
2 romaine lettuce hearts, chopped
60g black olives
10 baby plum tomatoes, halved

FOR THE DRESSING
1 garlic clove, grated
2 tbsp extra-virgin olive oil
Juice of 1 lemon
1 tsp Dijon mustard
Salt and black pepper

Preheat the oven to 180°C/350°F/gas mark 4.

Wrap the salmon fillets, either individually or together, in tinfoil, place them on a baking tray and bake in the oven for 15 minutes. The salmon should flake away easily when cooked.

Boil the baby potatoes in a saucepan of water with a pinch of salt for 15–20 minutes. Keeping the water in the pan, transfer the potatoes to a chopping board and cut them in half.

Return the water to the boil and cook the asparagus in the same saucepan for 2–3 minutes. Drain and place the asparagus in a bowl of cold water.

Cook the eggs in a fresh pan of boiling water for 6 minutes, then remove, and peel and quarter once cool.

To make the dressing, combine the garlic, olive oil, lemon juice and mustard in a small bowl with a sprinkle of salt and pepper, to taste. Whisk with a fork.

In a large bowl, toss the lettuce, olives, tomatoes, asparagus and potatoes in the dressing. Divide the salad between 2 bowls, flake the salmon fillets on top and add the chopped eggs.

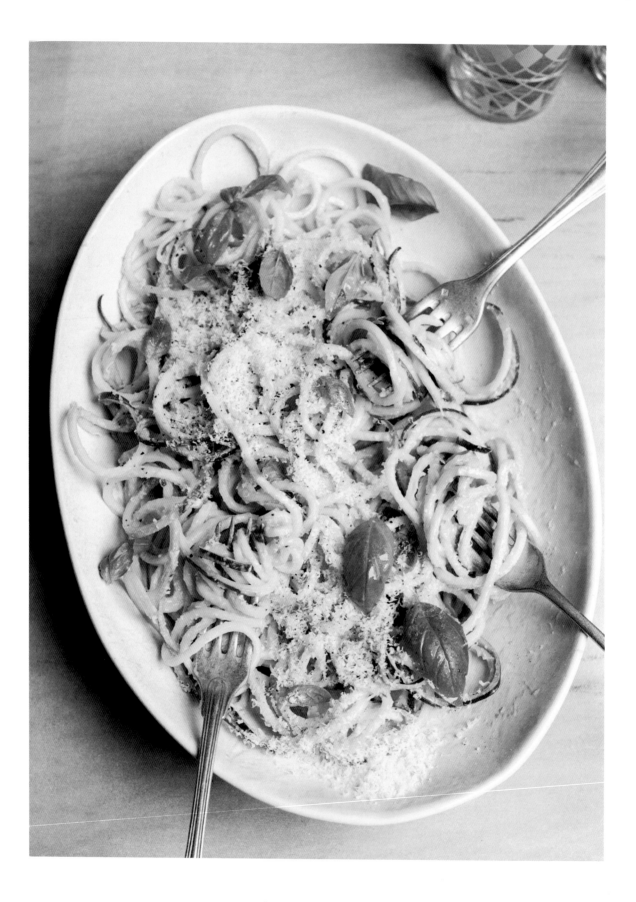

CREAMY AVOCADO + BASIL COURGETTI

One word – moreish. The dressing for this pasta alternative is so flavoursome, so creamy, and packed full of nutrients. Avocado is an awesome base for sauces because it's naturally creamy, full of healthy fats, low in sugar and very nutrient-dense. This is the meal I whip up on the weekend to impress friends and convince them that eating healthily isn't totally boring – or complicated. Serve it on its own as a lunch or light dinner, or as a side with salmon, chicken or feta cheese.

SERVES 2

2 large courgettes
1 ripe avocado
Juice of 1 small lemon
10 fresh basil leaves, plus a few more to garnish
2 garlic cloves
75ml water
2 tbsp grated Parmesan cheese, plus extra to garnish
2 tbsp pine nuts
Olive oil, for frying
Salt and black pepper

Make courgette noodles using a julienne peeler or spiraliser if you have one.

In a food processor, combine the rest of the ingredients and process until smooth and creamy.

If you prefer to eat the courgette raw, skip this step but otherwise, cook the courgette noodles for 1–2 minutes in a hot pan drizzled with olive oil.

Add the noodles to a large bowl and toss with the avocado pesto. Season with cracked pepper, a sprinkle of Parmesan, and some fresh basil.

TERIYAKI BEEF + ASIAN-STYLE BROCCOLI RICE

I love East Asian food, but you won't catch me picking up a takeaway at the local Chinese. Dishes from fast-food restaurants are generally pumped with MSG, flavourings, salt and trans fats, so they may leave you satisfied momentarily but soon after you're likely to feel sluggish and bloated. I would much rather spend a little more time making my own Asian-inspired meals that are nutritionally balanced, bursting with flavour, and that fill me with energy.

SERVES 4

500g lean beef steak, cut into chunks
½ tbsp coconut oil
1 lime, to serve

FOR THE BEEF MARINADE
1 garlic clove, grated
1 tbsp honey
1 tbsp Mirin
1 tbsp soy sauce*

FOR THE BROCCOLI RICE
40g cashews
1 broccoli head, cut into florets
½ tbsp coconut oil
1 red onion, diced
1 garlic clove, finely chopped
½ small red cabbage, shredded
1 red pepper, deseeded and sliced into strips
1 courgette, peeled into ribbons
2 spring onions, finely chopped

FOR THE SALAD DRESSING
Zest and juice of 1 lime
2 tbsp soy sauce*
½ tbsp coconut sugar**
1 tbsp olive oil

May be substituted with tamari.
**May be substituted with honey or brown sugar.*

Whisk together all the ingredients for the beef marinade in a small bowl. Place the beef chunks in a large ziplock bag and pour the marinade on top. Place the bag in the fridge for 1–3 hours.

Put a frying pan over a medium heat and add the cashews. Toast evenly, regularly shaking the pan, then remove and set aside.

Put the broccoli in a food processor and pulse until it resembles rice.

Heat the coconut oil in a large frying pan and fry the onion and garlic for 5 minutes. Add the broccoli rice to the pan and mix through. Sauté for 3–4 minutes.

Transfer the broccoli rice to a large bowl and add the red cabbage, pepper, courgette and spring onions.

To make the dressing, whisk together the ingredients and pour it over the salad. Set aside.

Fry the beef with the marinade on a griddle pan greased with the coconut oil. Cook for 5 minutes, turning, until cooked right through.

Serve the salad garnished with the toasted cashew nuts on top of the warm, sticky beef, with some lime on the side.

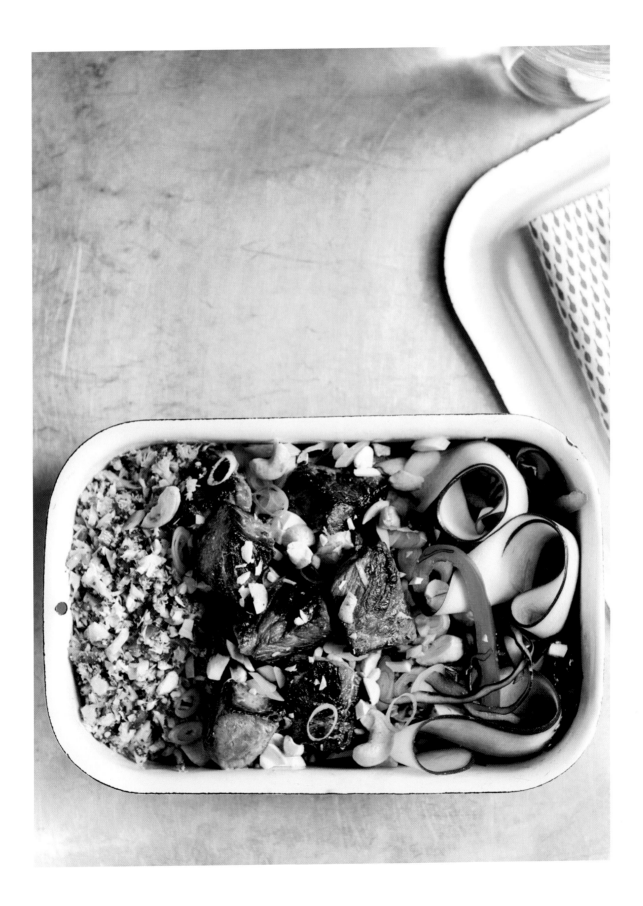

SWEET + SPICY CHICKEN BURGERS

Chicken mince makes for the easiest, leanest and juiciest burgers. I've added a sweet and spicy kick to this recipe to create a fun, tropical vibe. For the full Caribbean experience, add a slice of grilled pineapple to the burger and pop Bob Marley and the Wailers on!

MAKES 4 BURGERS

300g lean chicken mince
½ small red onion, finely diced
½ red chilli pepper, deseeded and
   finely chopped
60g sweetcorn
1 tbsp mango chutney
1 tbsp cornflour
1 tbsp coconut oil
Salt and black pepper

TO SERVE
Sweet potato chips, grilled slices
of pineapple, guacamole and salad

Using your hands, combine all the ingredients apart from the coconut oil together in a large bowl.

Form 4 even-sized burgers.

Place a frying pan over a medium–high heat and melt the coconut oil. Fry the burgers for about 5 minutes on each side until cooked right through.

Serve up with sweet potato chips, grilled pineapple, salad and guacamole.

PS... For a fun alternative, you can make these into meatball-sized balls and serve them in wraps.

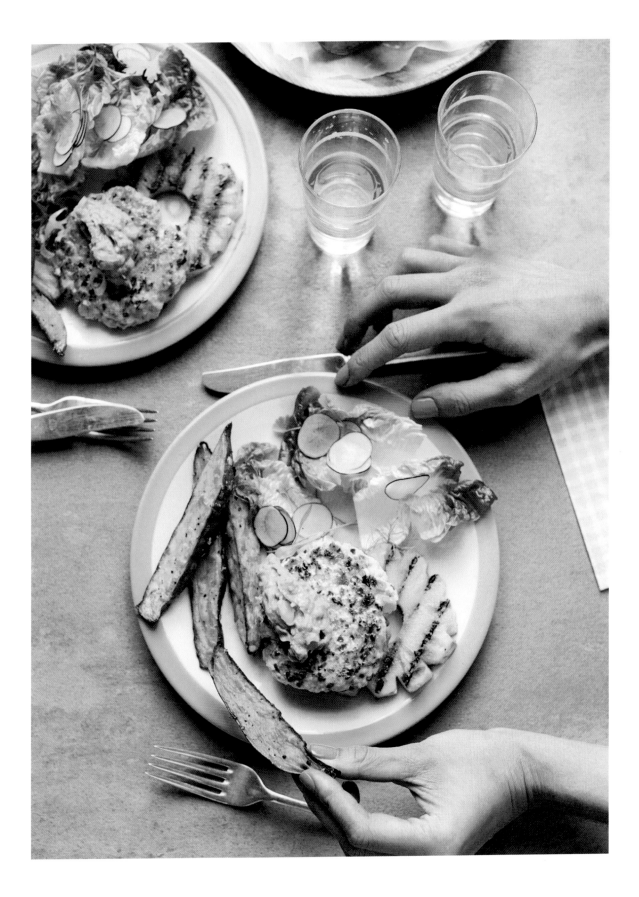

TURMERIC ROASTED CAULIFLOWER, CURRIED CHICKPEAS, + KALE SALAD

From cauliflower rice to cauliflower steaks, cauliflower seems to be the hottest vegetable on the block. It's an incredibly versatile vegetable which works as a great low-calorie substitute for starchy carbohydrates, such as rice and potato. I love roasting it in turmeric because of the incredible flavour, and colour, it gives the dish. Turmeric actually contains anti-inflammatory properties and has a long history of use in Ayurveda medicine – one extra reason to sprinkle it on your veggies.

SERVES 2 AS MAINS OR 4 AS SIDES

FOR THE KALE SALAD
1 tbsp extra-virgin olive oil
2 tbsp tahini, plus extra to drizzle
Juice of ½ lemon
1 garlic clove, minced or grated
1 tbsp water
¼ tsp salt
200g kale, shredded
½ red onion, finely sliced
2 tbsp mixed seeds

FOR THE ROASTED CAULIFLOWER
1 cauliflower head, cut into florets
½ tsp salt
2 tsp turmeric
1 tbsp extra-virgin olive oil

FOR THE CURRIED CHICKPEAS
½ tsp smoked paprika
½ tsp mild chilli powder
¼ tsp cumin
¼ tsp turmeric
¼ tsp salt
1 x 400g tin of chickpeas, rinsed and drained
1 tbsp extra-virgin olive oil

To make the dressing for the kale salad, whisk together the olive oil, tahini, lemon juice, garlic, water and salt. Pour it over the kale and massage for 2–3 minutes – massaging the kale softens the leaves and deepens the flavour of the salad. Cover with cling film and set aside. This step can be done several hours ahead of time.

Preheat the oven to 180°C/350°F/gas mark 4. Line a baking tray with tinfoil. Toss the cauliflower with the salt, turmeric and olive oil, and place on the baking tray. Bake for 30 minutes.

In a small bowl, combine the seasoning for the curried chickpeas. Add the spices to the chickpeas and gently toss. Heat the olive oil in a large pan and cook the chickpeas for 10 minutes.

Add the onion, seeds, roasted cauliflower and chickpeas to the kale salad and gently toss.

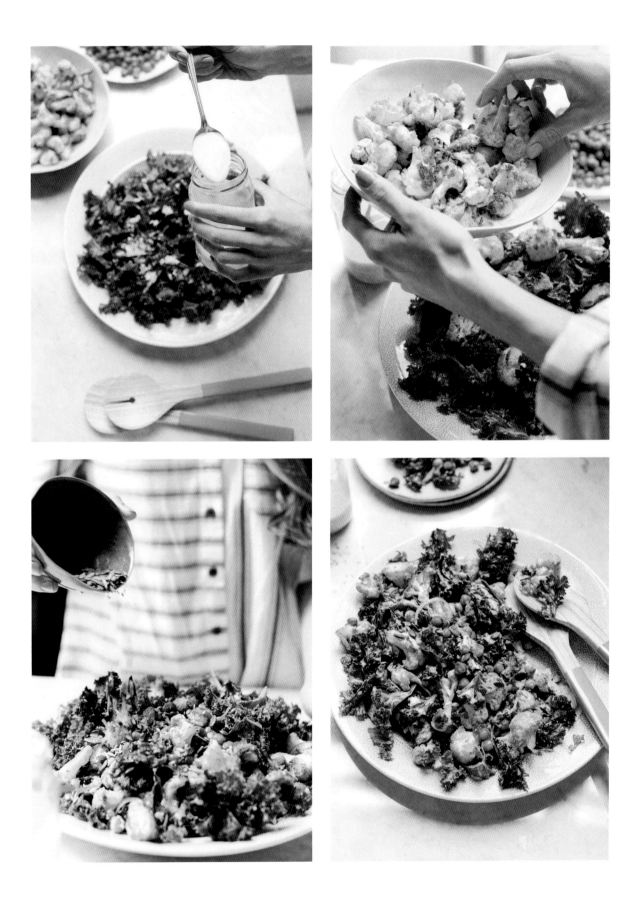

CRISPY CHICKEN GOUJONS WITH LETTUCE BOATS + CHUNKY SALSA

One of my favourite things to do is to recreate notoriously 'unhealthy' dishes as healthier, home-made versions. Chicken goujons are traditionally made by coating chicken strips in a flour- and egg-based batter, and then deep-fat frying them in vegetable oil until crispy – great for the tastebuds, but lethal for your heart and blood vessels (not to mention your waistline!) This recipe swaps the classic calorific batter for a naturally gluten-free, crunchy almond coating. For a heartier dish, serve this with crispy sweet potato fries.

SERVES 4

2 baby gem lettuce heads, leaves separated

FOR THE CHICKEN GOUJONS
50g whole almonds
¼ tsp cayenne pepper
¼ tsp garlic salt
½ tsp smoked paprika
4 chicken breasts, sliced into strips
1 tbsp coconut oil

FOR THE CHUNKY SALSA
1 avocado, diced
10 cherry tomatoes, quartered
1 red onion, diced
1 tbsp extra-virgin olive oil
Juice of ½ lemon
Salt and black pepper

To make the coating for the chicken goujons, place the almonds, cayenne pepper, garlic salt and smoked paprika in a blender and pulse several times until the nuts are chopped into smaller pieces, but not to a fine powder.

Place the chicken breast strips onto a plate and pour the coating on top. Using your hands, rub the coating into the chicken breasts until all the pieces are roughly coated.

Heat the coconut oil on a large griddle pan and fry the chicken strips for 5–10 minutes until cooked right through.

To make the chunky salsa, place the avocado, cherry tomatoes and red onion in a bowl. Pour over the olive oil and lemon juice. Mix well and season with a pinch of salt and pepper.

Serve each chicken strip in a lettuce leaf and top with a spoonful of salsa.

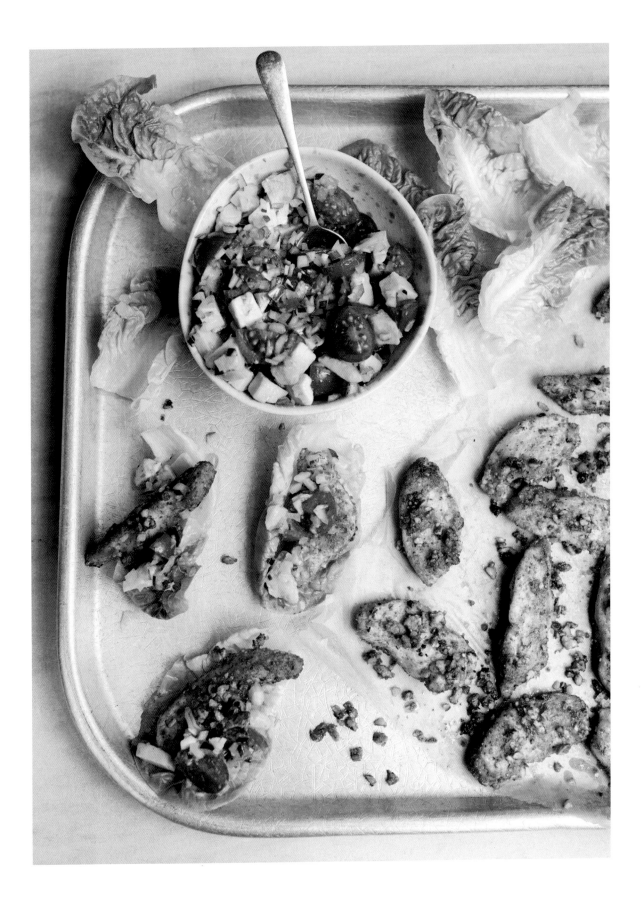

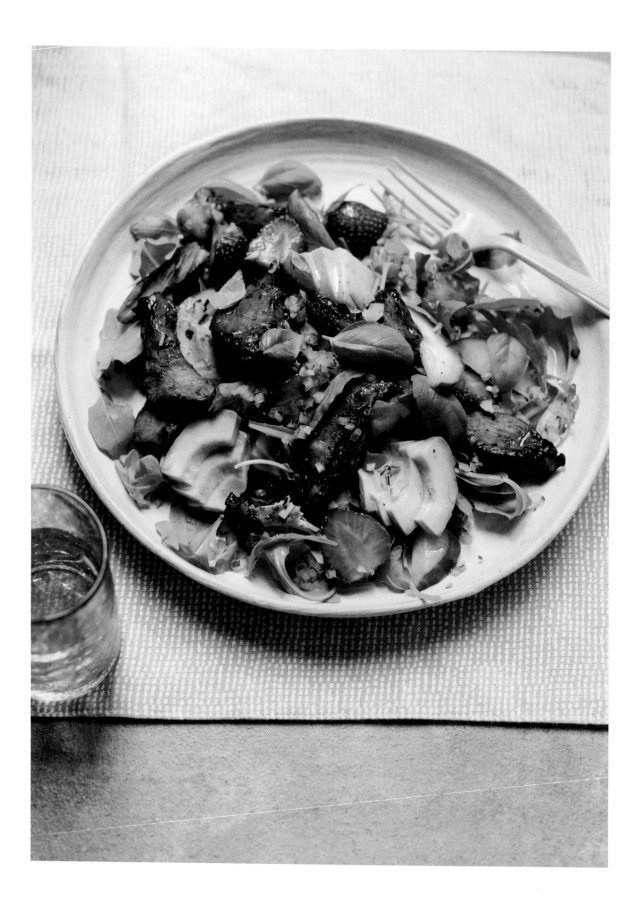

BALSAMIC CHICKEN WITH STRAWBERRY, AVOCADO + BASIL SALAD

This salad screams summer. It requires minimal ingredients, but each one provides an abundance of vitamins, minerals and flavours. I love the combination of the sweet strawberries and creamy avocado – I often pair them together on some rye bread with a little balsamic vinegar for a jazzy version of avo on toast. The grilled chicken rounds off this salad and boosts the protein content, but if you don't eat meat then try this with some feta, grilled halloumi or torn buffalo mozzarella.

SERVES 4

4 chicken breasts, cut into strips
4 tbsp balsamic vinegar

FOR THE SALAD
200g rocket leaves
2 avocados, diced
400g fresh strawberries, halved
1 red onion, finely chopped
1 cucumber, halved and sliced

FOR THE DRESSING
Handful of fresh basil leaves
    (about 10), plus extra to serve
2 tbsp extra-virgin olive oil
2 tbsp balsamic vinegar
Juice of 1 lemon
1 garlic clove
Salt and black pepper

Place the sliced chicken breasts and the balsamic vinegar in a ziplock bag in the fridge for at least 1–2 hours.

Preheat the oven to 200°C/400°F/gas mark 6 and bake the chicken with the balsamic vinegar for 25 minutes or until cooked right through.

To make the salad dressing, combine all the ingredients together in a blender. Season with salt and pepper.

Place the rocket, avocados, strawberries, onion and cucumber in a large mixing bowl. Pour the salad dressing on top and toss the salad until well coated.

Plate up the salad topped with the chicken and some fresh basil.

DECONSTRUCTED SUSHI SALAD

If you're a fan of sushi then you'll love this deconstructed sushi salad which takes just 15 minutes of prep and packs more nutritional punch than your typical takeaway sushi. For a vegetarian version, swap the smoked salmon for tofu or roasted sweet potato.

SERVES 2

120g brown rice
100g tender-stem broccoli
2 handfuls of spinach
150g smoked salmon
1 ripe avocado
2 spring onions, finely chopped
1 tbsp sesame seeds
1 nori seaweed sheet (optional)

FOR THE DRESSING
2 tbsp soy sauce or tamari
1 tsp honey
¼–½ tsp wasabi paste
Juice of ½ lime

Boil the rice for 25–30 minutes until soft, or for the length of time suggested on the packaging. Drain and set aside.

Steam or boil the broccoli for 5 minutes, then place in ice-cold water and drain.

Make the dressing by whisking all the ingredients together. Pour the dressing over the rice and mix well.

Take 2 separate bowls and place a handful of spinach in each. Divide the rice, smoked salmon, avocado and broccoli between the bowls.

Sprinkle with the spring onions and sesame seeds. If using the seaweed, cut it into small matchstick-sized strips with scissors and sprinkle over the top.

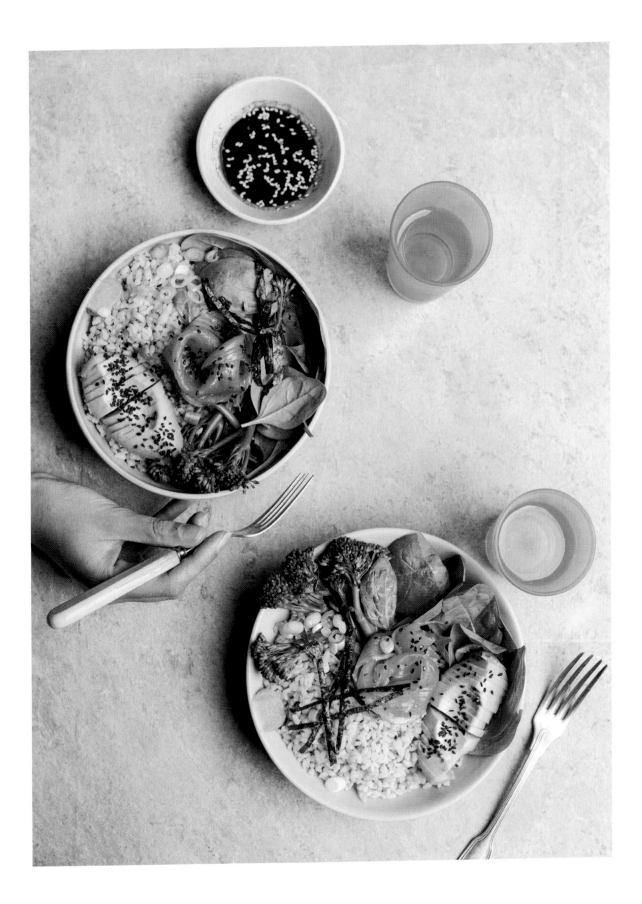

BEETROOT + FETA CAULI-RICE RISOTTO

White rice is long gone from my cupboard and although I love brown rice, it doesn't have the same texture that a refined rice gives to risotto – but cauli-rice does. The process is so simple, yet so delicious, as the cauliflower perfectly absorbs all the flavour, making it such a healthy replacement for refined, white rice. Not only does this dish taste amazing, but the beetroot gives it an incredible pink colour.

SERVES 2

2 large beetroots, cooked
120g Quark
2 tbsp balsamic vinegar
1 cauliflower head
1 tbsp coconut oil
½ red onion, diced
1 garlic clove, chopped
80g feta cheese, crumbled
Handful of fresh mint, finely chopped
Salt and black pepper

Using a blender or food processor, blend the beetroot, Quark and balsamic vinegar to form a creamy sauce.

Prepare the cauliflower rice by cutting the cauliflower head into 4, and then trimming out the inner core from each quarter. Break the cauliflower into smaller florets. Transfer the pieces to a food processor and pulse until the cauliflower has a cous cous-like texture.

Melt the coconut oil in a saucepan over a medium heat. Place the onion and garlic in the pan and fry gently for 5 minutes. Add the cauliflower rice to the pan and stir well. Season with salt and pepper to taste.

Stir in the beetroot sauce. Cook for 5–10 minutes until the temperature is warm right through.

Serve up on 2 plates and sprinkle with crumbled feta and mint.

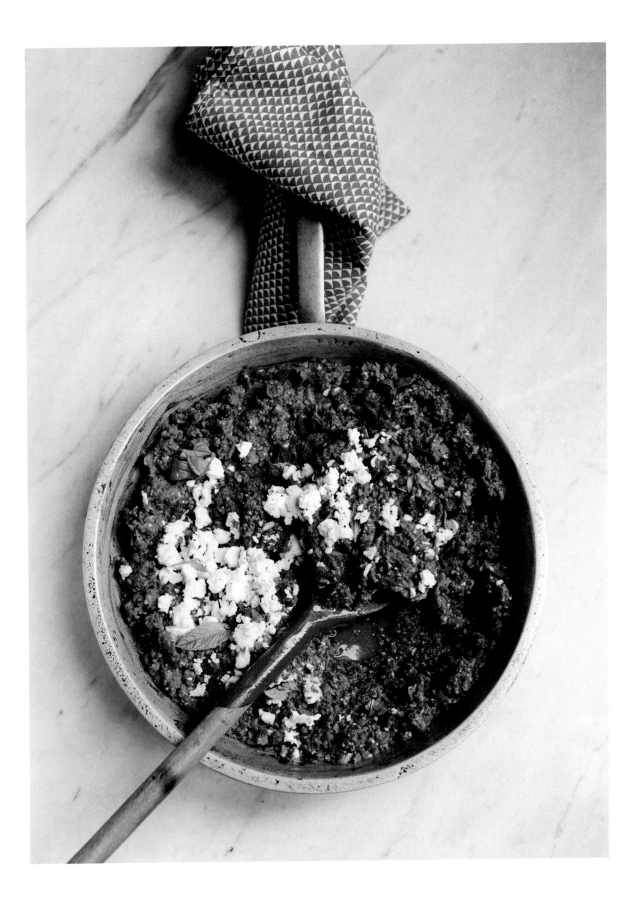

BAKED SWEET POTATO + SMOKY BAKED BEANS

As a university student, one of my favourite lazy meals was a baked potato with baked beans and lots of cheese.

Beans are a great source of protein and fibre, but tinned baked beans come in a sugary tomato sauce with added flavourings and preservatives. This recipe takes baked beans to a whole new level, in terms of nutrition and flavour, using a combination of kidney beans and butter beans in a home-made smoky tomato sauce. Serve it in a baked sweet potato for a healthy meat-free lunch, or on rye toast with poached eggs for a protein-packed breakfast!

SERVES 2

2 sweet potatoes
½ tbsp extra-virgin olive oil
½ tsp sea salt
1 tbsp coconut oil
1 garlic clove, finely chopped
½ red onion, diced
½ 240g tin of kidney beans, drained
½ 240g tin of butter beans, drained
½ 400g tin of chopped tomatoes
1 tsp smoked paprika
1 tsp chilli flakes
2 tbsp Greek yogurt
1 spring onion, chopped
Salt and black pepper

Preheat the oven to 200°C/400°F/gas mark 6. Pierce the sweet potatoes a few times with a fork, then cook them in the microwave on high for 8 minutes or until soft. Rub them with the olive oil and salt. Transfer them to a baking tray, put the tray in the oven and cook for 15–20 minutes until crispy.

To make the beans, melt the coconut oil in a saucepan. Add the garlic and onion, and fry for 2–3 minutes until translucent. Add the beans, chopped tomatoes, paprika and chilli flakes. Bring to a simmer and cook for a further 5–10 minutes until slightly reduced and thickened. Season with salt and pepper to taste.

Serve the sweet potatoes with the beans on top, a dollop of Greek yogurt and some spring onion.

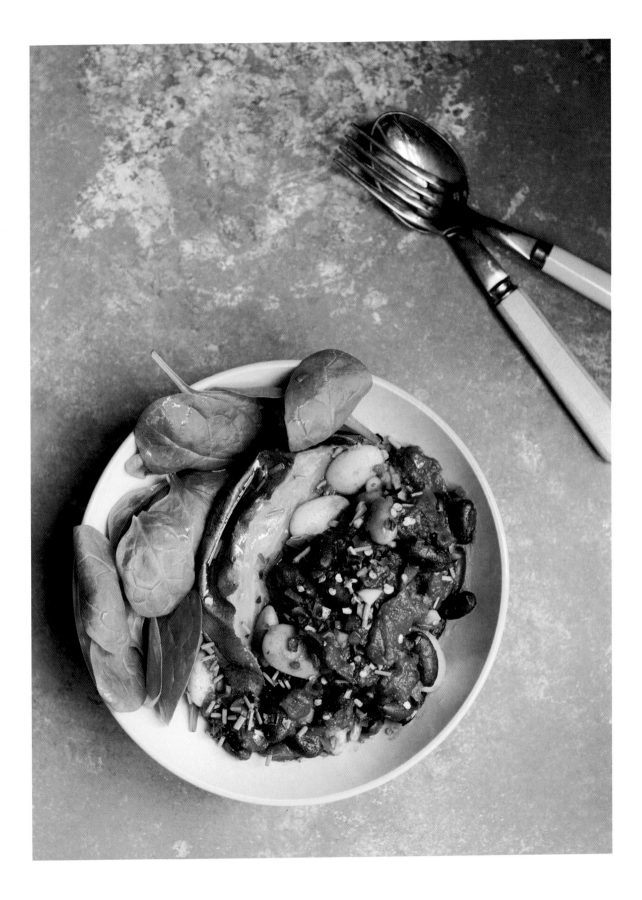

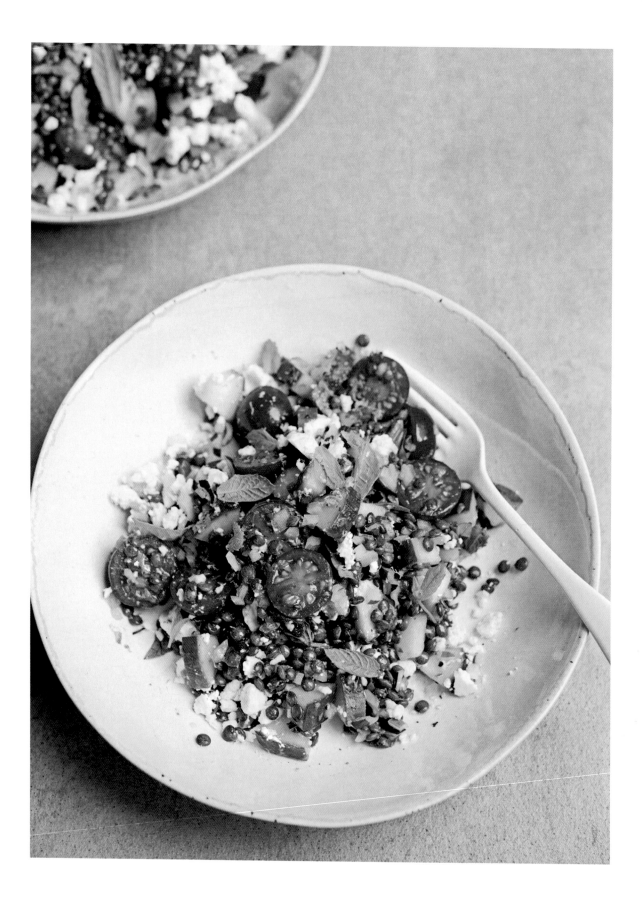

SUMMERY PUY LENTIL, FETA + MINT SALAD

One of my pet peeves is a bad salad. Shop-bought salads give salads a bad rep because they're so boring and empty with a few leaves of lettuce, a cherry tomato or two, and maybe – maybe – the odd piece of feta. I totally cannot justify spending money on something I could have made myself – only much better and for a fraction of the price.

If you still need to be convinced that salads can fill you up and satisfy you, then you need to try this recipe. The healthy fats from the feta cheese and oil-based dressing, coupled with the complex carbohydrates and fibre from the puy lentils and vegetables will keep you fuelled until dinner-time.

SERVES 2

120g puy lentils
500ml vegetable stock
½ cucumber
Handful of fresh mint, roughly
  chopped
10 cherry tomatoes, halved
½ red onion, finely chopped
1 lemon
1 tbsp extra-virgin olive oil
¼ tsp of salt
100g feta cheese, to serve
Black pepper

Rinse the lentils in cold water, drain and place them in a saucepan. Pour the stock on top of the lentils. Bring to the boil and reduce to a simmer for 25 minutes. Drain and set aside to cool for at least 60 minutes.

Halve the cucumber lengthways and remove the seeds. Then halve each piece again lengthways so that you have 4 long pieces. Chop the pieces into small chunks. Place the cucumber, mint, tomatoes, red onion and lentils in a large mixing bowl.

Grate the zest off the lemon and add it to the mixture. Cut the lemon in half and squeeze the juice of 1 half on top.

Drizzle the olive oil on top, and season with the salt and pepper. Toss.

Serve in 2 bowls and crumble half the cheese over each bowl.

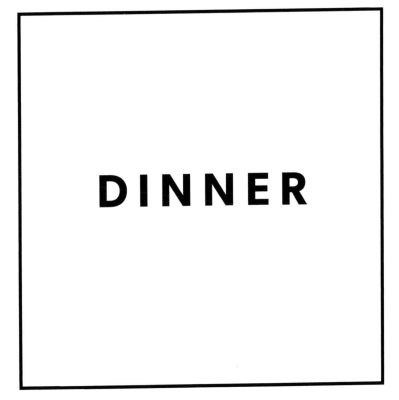
DINNER

My recipes for dinner tend to be super-quick and super-simple.

There is nothing I love more than coming home after a long day, kicking my shoes off and cooking something really delicious for dinner! The reality is, most of us just don't have hours to spend in the evening preparing and cooking dinner. I get it. That's why my recipes tend to be super-quick and super-simple, without sacrificing nutrition or taste.

I've included some of my favourite healthy 'fakeaways' for those Friday nights when you're craving something that feels a little bit more like a treat! For a night in with friends or family (particularly my sister, pictured with me here), I love to knock up a big platter of loaded sweet potato nachos and chilli (page 192) or rice paper chicken rolls with peanut butter dipping sauce (page 178) for everyone to nibble on.

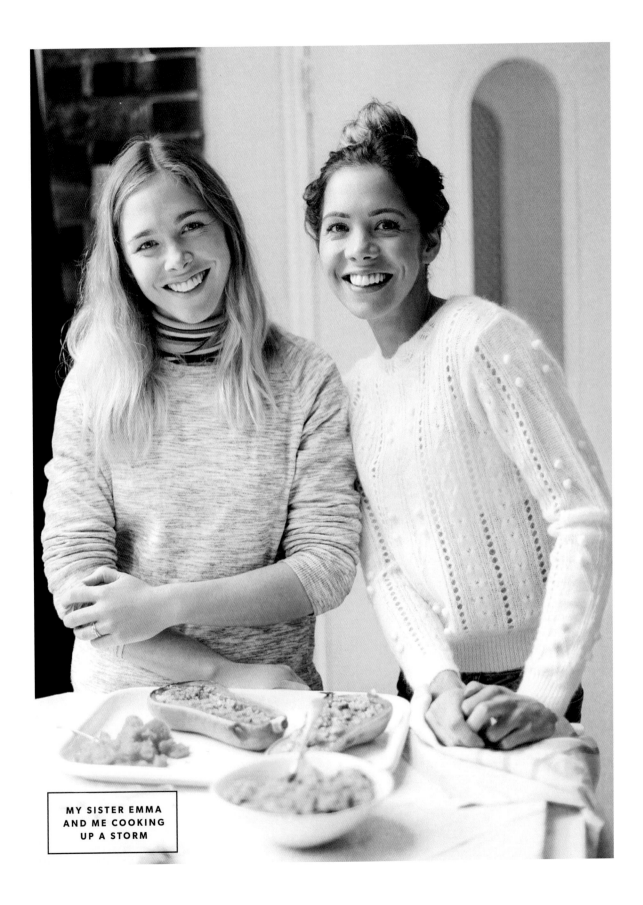

MY SISTER EMMA
AND ME COOKING
UP A STORM

STICKY SOY ROASTED SALMON + AUBERGINE

This is my favourite way to eat salmon fillets – especially when I remember to let them marinate overnight and let the flavours soak right in, leaving the most tender, flaky and flavoursome salmon that you will ever try. The marinade is really simple to make, using basic ingredients that you probably have sitting in your cupboard already.

SERVES 2

2 tbsp soy sauce*
2 tbsp honey
1 garlic clove, grated
2 fresh salmon fillets
1 aubergine
1 tbsp olive oil
2 spring onions, finely chopped
120g tender-stem broccoli
1 tbsp coconut oil
Juice of ½ lemon
150g edamame beans
Coriander, to garnish
Salt and black pepper

May be substituted with tamari.

In a small bowl, combine 1 tablespoon of the soy sauce, 1 tablespoon of the honey and the garlic.

Place the salmon fillets in a ziplock bag and pour the soy marinade on top. Seal and store the salmon in the fridge overnight or for several hours to allow the salmon to soak up the flavours.

Preheat the oven to 180°C/350°F/gas mark 4. Cut the aubergine in half lengthways and lightly score each half with a knife in a criss-cross pattern. Place the halves on a sheet of tinfoil on a baking tray.

Combine the olive oil and the remaining soy sauce and honey in a small bowl, and pour the mixture on top of the aubergine.

Bake in the oven for 25 minutes. Spoon any marinade in the base of the tray on top of the aubergine and sprinkle the spring onion on top, before placing the tray back in the oven for another 10–15 minutes. Place the salmon fillets on a sheet of tinfoil on a baking tray and bake in the oven alongside the aubergine and spring onion.

Sauté the tender-stem broccoli in the coconut oil and lemon juice in a hot frying pan for 5–8 minutes. Toss in the edamame beans and fry for another 2 minutes. Sprinkle with coriander and season with salt and pepper to taste.

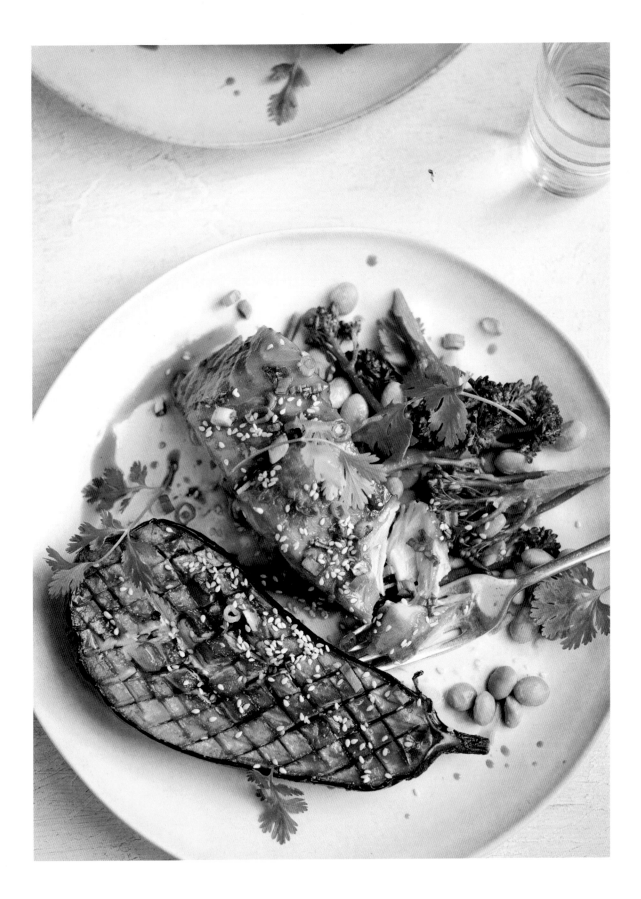

PARMA HAM WRAPPED COD FILLETS + MEDITERRANEAN VEGETABLES

Cod is an amazing source of lean protein, vitamins and minerals, but let's be honest, it can taste pretty bland when it's cooked on its own. By coating the cod in pesto and wrapping it in Parma ham, it seals in the juices and adds so much more flavour to the fish.

SERVES 2

FOR THE COD

2 tsp classic green pesto

2 cod fillets

2 basil leaves

4 slices of Parma ham or
  prosciutto

FOR THE MEDITERRANEAN VEGETABLES

2 tbsp extra-virgin olive oil

Juice of 1 lemon

1 tbsp balsamic vinegar

1 garlic clove, grated

10 basil leaves

10 cherry tomatoes

1 courgette, halved and sliced

2 bell peppers, seeds removed,
  chopped

1 red onion, roughly chopped

8 baby potatoes

Salt and black pepper

Preheat the oven to 180°C/350°F/gas mark 4. Make the dressing for the vegetables by combining the olive oil, lemon juice, balsamic vinegar, garlic and basil leaves in a blender.

Place the cherry tomatoes, courgette, peppers, and red onion in a large roasting tin. Pour the dressing over the vegetables and toss. Season with salt and pepper. Roast the vegetables for 25–30 minutes.

Prepare the cod fillets by spreading a teaspoon of pesto over each fillet, topped with a basil leaf. Wrap each fillet in 2 slices of ham.

Place the potatoes in a small saucepan of water. Bring the water to the boil, lower the heat and simmer for 5–10 minutes until the potatoes are just tender. Drain the potatoes and slice in half.

Take the vegetables out of the oven and add the potatoes, tossing them with the vegetables and the dressing. Make a space amongst the vegetables and place the 2 cod fillets in the roasting tin. Spoon some of the juices from the vegetables on top of the cod fillets. Return the entire tray to the oven for another 15 minutes.

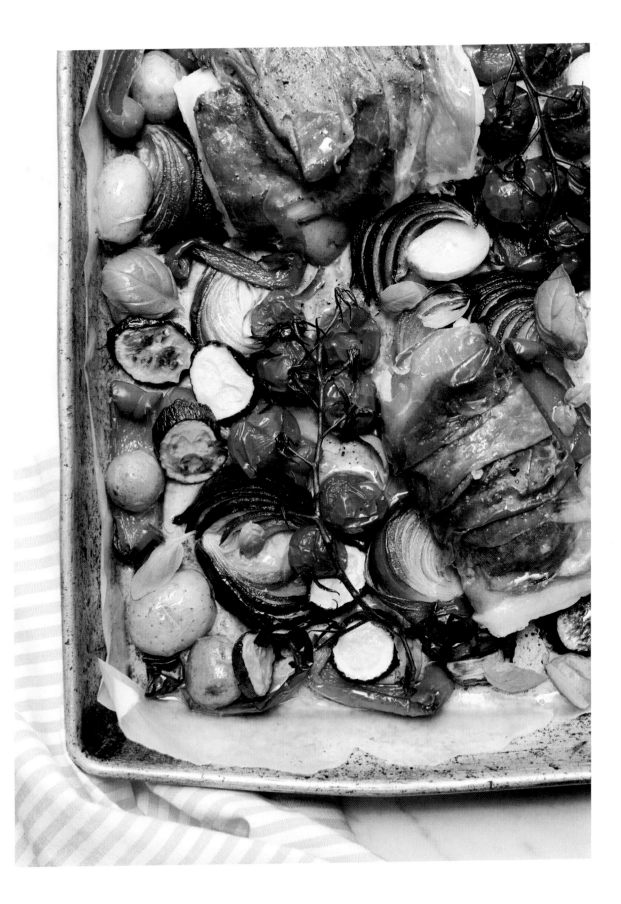

HEALTHY BANGERS + MASH

Bangers and mash – another traditional comfort food from home. Like many British and Irish dishes, it involves meat and spuds. This healthy twist is packed with protein and low in fat, easy to make, and loaded with flavour, it's the perfect dish for a cosy night in. I've used chicken sausages in this recipe because they are generally a leaner meat than pork, with a higher protein content per serving.

SERVES 3

6 chicken sausages
½ butternut squash, peeled and chopped
2 carrots, peeled and diced
2 parsnips, peeled and diced
50ml almond milk
1 tbsp butter
1 tbsp coconut oil
1 red onion, sliced into rings
2 tbsp balsamic vinegar
1 tbsp cornflour
250ml vegetable stock
Salt and black pepper

Preheat the oven to 180°C/350°F/gas mark 4. Bake the sausages for 30 minutes until golden.

Place the squash, carrots and parsnips in a saucepan of water. Bring the water to the boil for 10 minutes until soft. Drain in a colander and return the vegetables to the pot. Add the milk and butter, and mash. Add salt and pepper to taste.

Melt the coconut oil in a frying pan over a medium–high heat. Add the onion and fry for 5 minutes. Next, add the balsamic vinegar.

In a separate bowl, whisk together the cornflour and stock, adding the stock slowly.

Add the stock and cornflour to the onions. Bring to the boil and simmer for 5 minutes, until it thickens to a gravy.

Serve the root mash topped with sausages and pour the sweet onion gravy over the top.

SALMON PIE WITH CAULIFLOWER MASH

This lighter version of the classic fish pie is one of my favourite dinners to make when I have a little more time on my hands. It's really versatile so you can use any fish you wish, or even a combination of different fish, such as cod, haddock, salmon and prawns. The creamy cauliflower mash makes this a hearty but healthy dish, loaded with fibre, vitamins and minerals.

SERVES 4

1½ cauliflower heads
50g light cream cheese
4 spring onions, thinly sliced
160g frozen peas
1 tbsp coconut oil
1 small white onion, diced
1 leek, sliced
2 garlic cloves, chopped or grated
500g salmon boneless fillet, separated into chunks
250ml almond milk or skimmed milk
1 tbsp cornflour
2 tsp dill
Salt and black pepper

Preheat the oven to 180°C/350°F/gas mark 4.

Cut the cauliflower into florets and boil for 10 minutes until soft. Drain, add the cream cheese, salt and pepper, and blend using a hand blender. Stir in the spring onions and set aside.

Boil the peas in a small pan of water or in the microwave, according to the packet instructions.

Heat the coconut oil in a large pan, add the onion, leek and garlic, and cook for 5 minutes until soft. Add the salmon and the peas, and cook for a further 5 minutes.

In a small bowl, whisk the milk and cornflour together until well combined. Add them to the pan with the salmon and vegetables, and bring everything to the boil. Allow to simmer for 4-5 minutes as the sauce thickens. Season with dill, salt and pepper.

Transfer the mixture to an ovenproof pyrex dish and top with the cauliflower mash.

Bake in the oven for 25 minutes until golden on the top and bubbling at the sides.

Best served with fresh green beans.

SMOKY CHICKEN + CHICKPEA STEW WITH ROASTED BUTTERNUT SQUASH WEDGES

As a child, the word 'stew' would make me squirm but now I make stews all the time. I love spooning this stew into big bowls for a super-easy, filling meal to have after a long day at work, or to make in batches ahead of time for weekday lunches. I serve it with butternut squash wedges to mop up the extra liquid but it also works amazingly with quinoa or rice.

FOR THE CHICKEN + CHICKPEA STEW

500g chicken breasts, diced
Juice of 1 lime
1 tsp smoked paprika
1 tsp chilli powder
1 tbsp coconut oil
1 red onion, diced
2 garlic cloves, finely chopped
1 jar of roasted red peppers, drained and sliced
1 x 400g tin of chopped tomatoes
1 x 400g tin of chickpeas, rinsed and drained
Salt and black pepper

FOR THE ROASTED BUTTERNUT SQUASH

1 tbsp coconut oil
1 tsp cinnamon
1 tsp smoked paprika
1 butternut squash
Salt and black pepper

TIP: *Make ahead and refrigerate for up to three days for healthy lunches or last-minute dinners.*

Preheat the oven to 200°C/400°F/gas mark 6.

Melt a tablespoon of coconut oil for 20 seconds in the microwave. Stir in the cinnamon and paprika.

Halve the squash cross-wise and scoop out the seeds. Cut the squash into 1cm thick half rings. Place the squash in a large mixing bowl and drizzle the coconut oil mixture on top, tossing it all with your hands to ensure all the squash is coated. Sprinkle some salt and pepper on top.

Arrange the squash on a large baking tray lined with greaseproof paper. (You may need 2 trays.) Bake in the oven for 45 minutes, turning once to cook both sides, until they soften and turn golden.

Place the chicken breasts in a large mixing bowl with the lime juice, smoked paprika and chilli powder.

Put a large saucepan over a medium heat with 1 tablespoon of coconut oil. Add the onion and garlic, and sauté for 2–3 minutes before adding the chicken. Fry for 10 minutes until the chicken is golden and cooked right through.

Add the peppers, tomatoes and chickpeas to the saucepan. Stir well and bring to the boil for a minute before reducing the heat. Cover and allow to simmer for 15–20 minutes. Season with a sprinkle of salt and pepper.

Serve the stew in bowls or on plates with the roasted butternut squash.

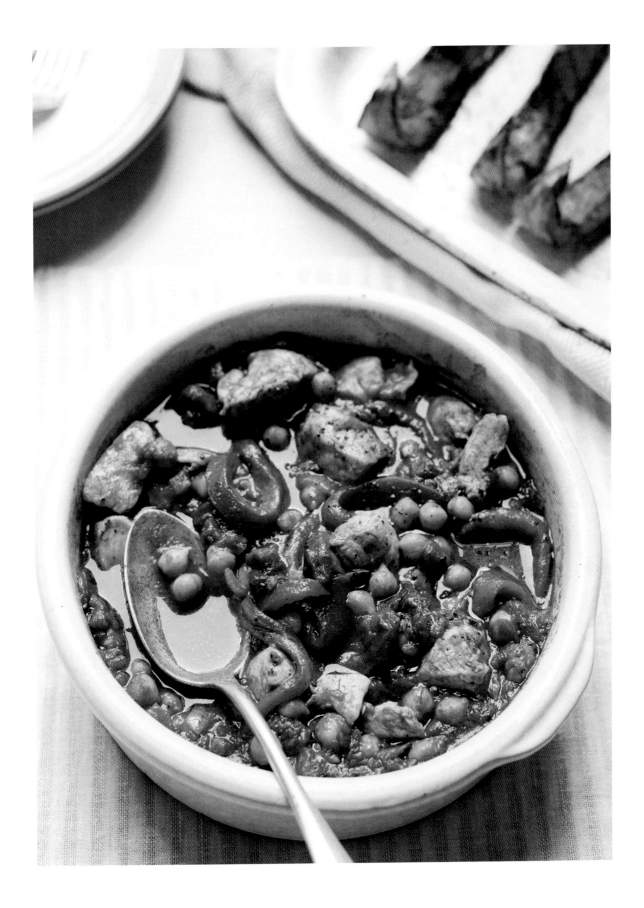

HEALTHY HOME-MADE PIZZA IN A FLASH

Home-made pizza is an art – a very delicious, time-consuming art. For those of us with busy lifestyles (essentially all of us), there isn't the time to be slogging away in the kitchen making pizza dough from scratch. I often find myself craving a pizza on the weekend, and sometimes I will use a tortilla wrap as the base or I'll make my own. This pizza recipe calls for a handful of ingredients and it takes less than 5 minutes to make. I've given you a few ideas for toppings but feel free to try whatever weird and wonderful combinations your heart desires. My personal favourite? Goat's cheese, red onion, fresh rocket and a drizzle of balsamic vinegar.

SERVES 1

4 large free-range egg whites
2 tbsp coconut flour
¼ tsp dried oregano
¼ tsp dried basil
2 tbsp passata or tomato purée
Melted coconut oil, for greasing

FOR THE TOPPINGS
Classic margherita: torn mozzarella, sundried tomatoes and fresh basil
Handful of black olives, crumbled feta cheese, cherry tomatoes and fresh basil
Rocket, red onion, goat's cheese and a drizzle of balsamic vinegar
Parma ham, Parmesan cheese and fresh rocket
Torn chicken, red bell peppers, jalepeño peppers and mozzarella
Roasted aubergine, courgette, pepper, red onion and mozzarella

In a large mixing bowl, whisk the egg whites.

In a separate bowl, sift the coconut flour and add the dried herbs. Pour the dry mixture into the egg whites and whisk for 2–3 minutes until all the clumps are removed and the mixture is smooth.

Place a large non-stick frying pan greased with coconut oil over a medium–high heat. Pour the mixture into the pan and shape into a pizza. Reduce the heat and allow it to cook for 4–5 minutes on each side.

Place the pizza base on a flat baking tray lined with tinfoil. Spread the passata over the base and add your favourite toppings.

Place under a hot grill for 5 minutes until the cheese has melted. If you're using uncooked vegetables as toppings, you can bake the pizza in an oven preheated to 180°C/350°F/gas mark 4 for 15–20 minutes to soften the toppings and melt the cheese.

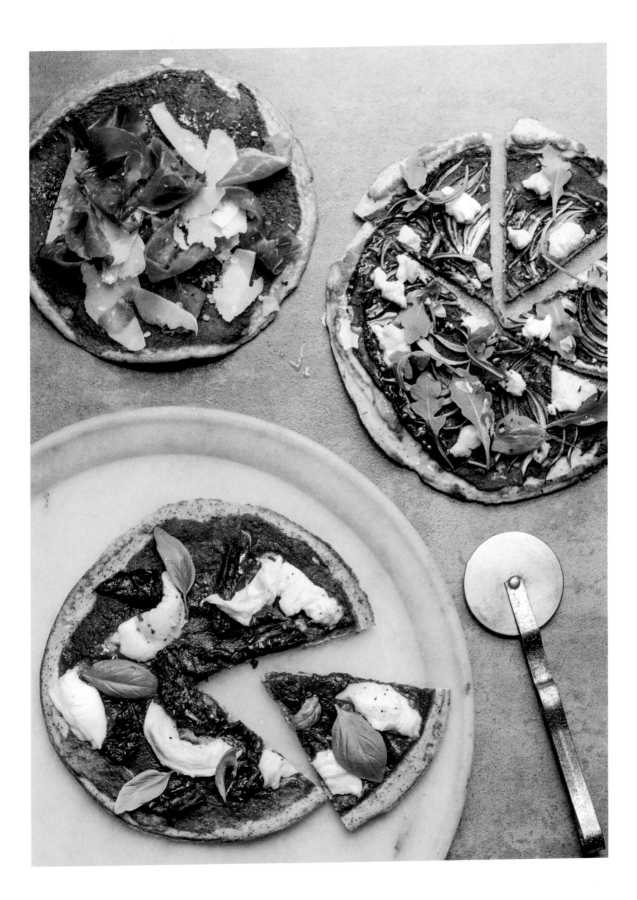

RICE PAPER CHICKEN ROLLS WITH PEANUT BUTTER DIPPING SAUCE

I first tried this recipe as an experiment when I was trying to impress my boyfriend on date night. It is such a fun dish to make with a friend, or your partner, and it encourages everyone to get involved and roll up their sleeves. The rice paper wraps are really light and combined with the raw vegetables, this dish is much lighter and fresher than your classic Mexican chicken fajita. For a veggie alternative, swap the chicken breast for avocado.

SERVES 2 AS MAINS OR 4 AS STARTERS

8 spring roll wrappers (rice paper wraps)
¼ red cabbage, shredded
¼ cucumber, cut into matchsticks
1 red pepper, cut into matchsticks
½ mango, cut into matchsticks
2 spring onions, thinly sliced
2 chicken breasts, cooked and shredded

FOR THE PEANUT DIPPING SAUCE
3 tbsp smooth peanut butter
1 tbsp coconut sugar
2 tbsp water
1 tbsp soy sauce*

May be substituted with tamari.

Fill a large bowl with warm water. Immerse 1 spring roll wrapper in the water until slightly softened (for about 10–15 seconds). Remove and spread the wrapper out onto a plastic chopping board. Repeat with all the wrappers.

Place some of each of the ingredients horizontally at the bottom or centre of a wrap, packing them as tightly together as possible. Fold in the right and left edges of the wrap. Take the bottom of the wrap and roll it upwards, taking the ingredients with it. Try to wrap them as tightly as possible, then leave the wrap sealed-side down. Place the roll on a plate and repeat.

To make the dressing, blend or whisk the ingredients together until smooth. Pour into a small serving dish and serve on the side to dip the wraps in.

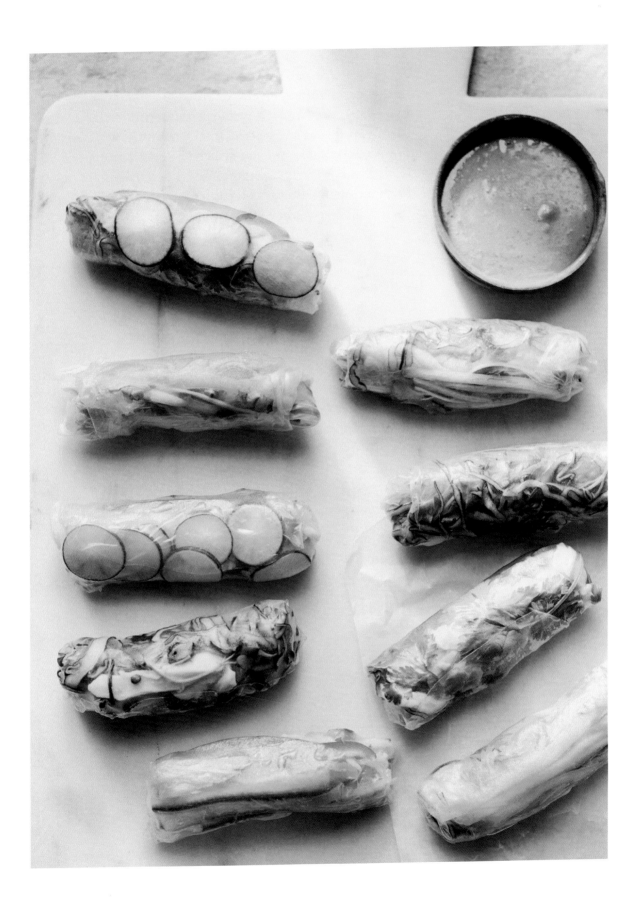

VEGGIE-LOADED BEEF BOLOGNESE WITH COURGETTI

Growing up, Bolognese was made at least once a week. It was one of mine and my dad's favourites. My mum had her recipe nailed and she would serve it with fresh Parmesan cheese and warm garlic bread. This recipe is my own, super-chunky version of a classic beef Bolognese loaded with lots of good vegetables. The minced beef can be substituted for any other minced meat, or cooked lentils for a meat-free version.

SERVES 4

1 onion, diced
2 garlic cloves, finely chopped
1 tbsp coconut oil
400g lean steak mince meat
1 tsp dried oregano
1 tsp dried basil
1 courgette, diced
1 red pepper, chopped
1 yellow pepper, chopped
200g mushrooms, sliced
30g black olives, chopped
1 x 500g carton of passata
3 tbsp of tomato purée
150ml beef or vegetable stock.
Bunch of fresh basil leaves,
    roughly chopped
4 courgettes

TO SERVE
Freshly grated Parmesan
(*optional*)

In a large pan, sauté the onions and garlic in the coconut oil over a medium heat until soft.

Add the mince and dried herbs, and cook for 5–10 minutes until brown. Remove the pan from the heat, drain off any excess water and transfer everything to a large saucepan.

Add the vegetables, passata, tomato purée and stock. Bring to the boil and reduce to a simmer for 20–30 minutes until the sauce starts to thicken. The longer you let it simmer, the richer the sauce will become. Turn off the heat and stir in the basil.

To make the courgetti, spiralise the courgettes if you have a spiraliser or peel them into thin ribbons using a julienne peeler.

Serve the Bolognese on top of the courgetti with a sprinkle of Parmesan, if using.

PS... If you're not a fan of chunky vegetables, blend the vegetables with the passata and tomato purée until smooth.

MUM'S FRUITY CURRY

I have to thank my mum for the recipe for this sweet and mildly spiced curry. I absolutely love curries but I'm a total weakling when it comes to hot dishes. The fruit in this curry tones down the heat so you can savour all the spices – without having to chase every mouthful with a gulp of cold water. This dish works well when cooking for a group as the recipe can be doubled up and made the night before, then slowly heated back up over a low heat or in a slow cooker when it's time to eat. I actually prefer this the next day after the chicken has soaked up all the flavour from the peaches and curry spices – YUM!

SERVES 4–5

1 tbsp coconut oil
1 onion, diced
500g chicken breast, diced
2 tbsp hot mango chutney
1 apple, diced
1 x 411g tin of peaches in juice, drained
2 tbsp mild curry paste
1 tsp of curry powder
300ml chicken stock
100ml light coconut milk
50g raisins

In a large frying pan, heat the coconut oil and fry the onion until soft and translucent. Add the chicken and cook for 10 minutes until cooked right through.

Add the chutney, apple, peaches, curry paste and curry powder and stir them into the mixture.

Pour in the stock, bring to the boil and simmer over a low heat for 20–25 minutes, stirring occasionally. The liquid should reduce down.

Add the coconut milk and raisins, and allow to simmer for another 5 minutes over a low heat.

Serve with rice or roasted butternut squash.

STEAK WITH BALSAMIC ROASTED CARROTS + PARSNIPS

Many of us tend to avoid red meat when we're trying to be healthier because of the way it is portrayed in the media – as unhealthy and even dangerous.

We really shouldn't exclude this nutritious food from our diet. Red meat is packed with protein, which is critical for muscle growth and recovery, and is also high in iron and vitamin B-12, which is vital for healthy red blood cells, and our brain and nervous system. Red meat has only come under the spotlight because of the health concerns surrounding processed meats, i.e. meat that has been smoked, cured, salted or preserved in some other way. We don't need to stop eating processed meat altogether but when buying red meat, it's better to choose the best quality, from animals that have been grass-fed and raised organically, without drugs and hormones. These cuts of meat are slightly more expensive but if you're only having steak once a week, or once every two weeks, then it's really worth the extra few pennies.

SERVES 2

3 tbsp coconut oil
3 tbsp balsamic vinegar
3 carrots, sliced lengthways
2 parsnips, sliced lengthways
1 red onion, sliced into rings
2 fillet steaks (grass-fed if possible)
100g spinach
1 tbsp butter
Salt and black pepper

Preheat the oven to 200°C/400°F/gas mark 6.

Melt 1 tablespoon of the coconut oil in the microwave for 20 seconds. Add 2 tablespoons of the balsamic vinegar and a pinch of salt and pepper. Toss with the carrots and parsnips in a large bowl. Bake on a flat baking tray for 40 minutes, turning once or twice in between.

Place a large griddle pan over a medium heat with another tablespoon of coconut oil. Fry the red onion for 2–3 minutes, reduce the heat and add the remaining balsamic vinegar. Stir.

Set aside the onions, and use the same pan to cook the steaks for 3–5 minutes on each side, depending on taste. Transfer the steaks to plates.

Put the spinach in a saucepan with the butter and a little seasoning, then cover and place over a medium heat for 1 minute or until just wilted. Serve with the steak and vegetables.

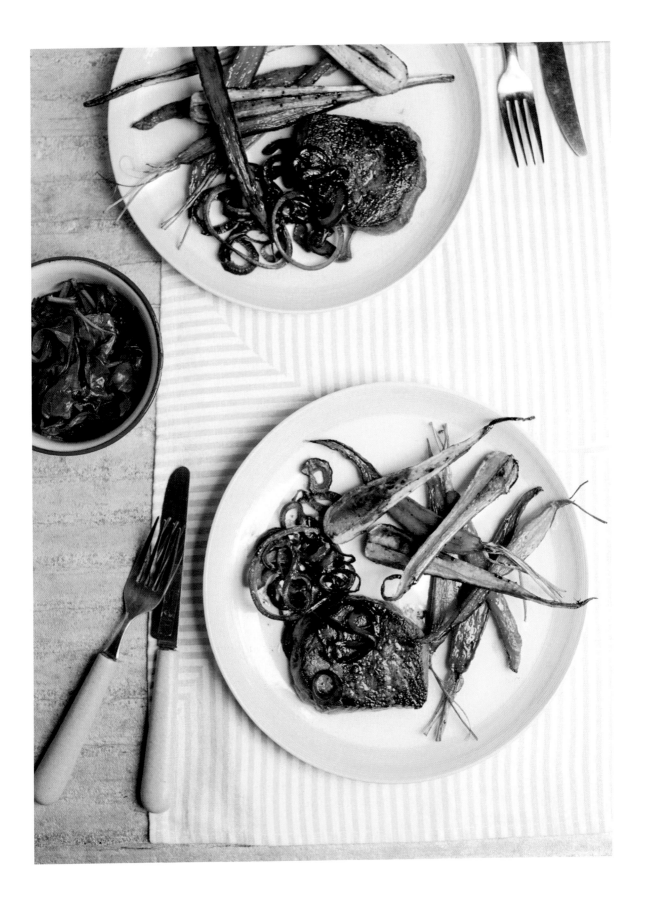

FISH 'N' CHIPS: CRUSTED COD, MINTED MUSHY PEAS + PARSNIP FRIES

There's nothing quite like chip shop fish and chips wrapped up in brown paper with lots of salt and vinegar. However, your average portion of fish 'n' chips totals close to 1,000kcal, and a whopping amount of trans fats and salt. So in true Food Medic style, I've given this classic dish a healthy makeover by swapping the usual batter for a crispy almond coating and the greasy, fried potato chips for oven-roasted parsnip fries – saving you more than half the calories. Don't worry, you're not just losing calories here – you're increasing the nutritional content of the meal and also amping up the flavour.

SERVES 2

FOR THE COD
1 free-range egg
1 tbsp ground almonds
25g flaked almonds
1 tsp dried dill
2 cod fillets
Cracked black pepper

FOR THE MINTED MUSHY PEAS
300g frozen peas
1 tbsp grass-fed butter
6 mint leaves

FOR THE PARSNIP FRIES
2 large parsnip, peeled and sliced into chips
1 tbsp coconut oil
2 rosemary sprigs, chopped
Salt and black pepper

Preheat the oven to 200°C/400°F/gas mark 6.

Place the parsnip chips in a large bowl. Melt the coconut oil in the microwave for 15–20 seconds and pour it over the chips. Add the rosemary, salt and pepper, and toss the ingredients together. Place the seasoned fries on a flat baking tray and bake them for 20–25 minutes, turning them once or twice to ensure all sides are golden and crisp.

To make the crusted cod fillets, first beat the egg with a fork in a shallow bowl. In another bowl, combine the ground almonds, flaked almonds, dill and a sprinkle of pepper. Spread the mixture onto a plate. Take the cod fillets and dip them, 1 at a time, into the egg mixture and then into the almond coating. It might not stick easily, so you may have to press the fillets into the almonds. When the parsnips are halfway through cooking, remove them from the oven and add the fillets on the baking tray and bake for 10–15 minutes until the crust is golden.

Boil the peas in a small saucepan according to the packet instructions and drain. Place the peas back in the saucepan with the butter and sauté for 1 minute until the butter melts and coats the peas entirely. Remove the pan from the heat, season and add the mint. Using a hand blender, purée the peas roughly so that some texture remains in the dish.

Serve up the fish with the mushy peas and crispy parsnip fries – for an extra fish shop feel, wrap the fries in newspaper!

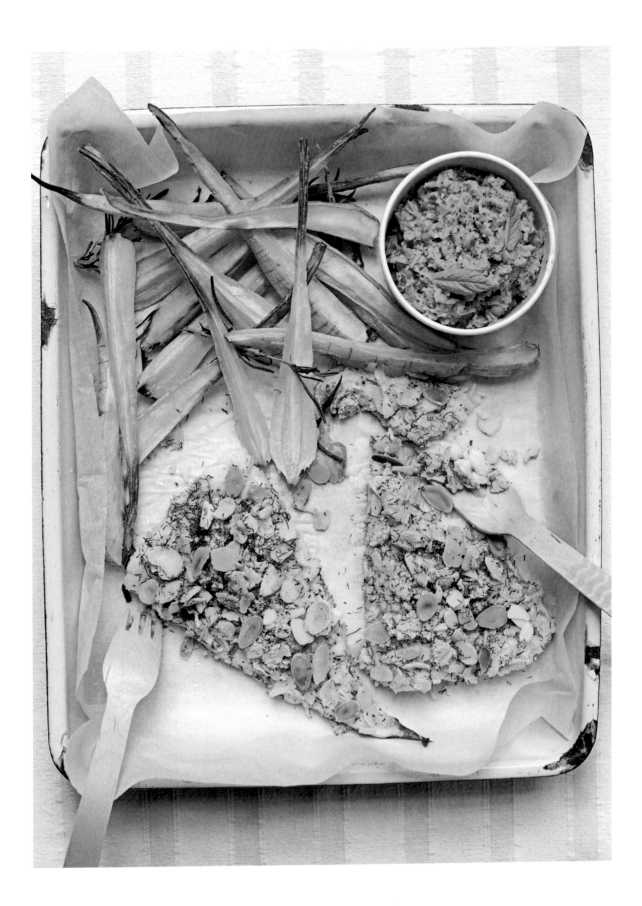

GREEK LAMB MEATBALL WRAPS WITH TZATZIKI SAUCE

Lamb mince makes the best meatballs in my opinion, but you can substitute the meat for beef, turkey or chicken mince. There are also so many ways you can eat them – in a wrap, on a salad, on courgette noodles, or simply on their own off a toothpick as a quick, high-protein snack. My favourite way to eat them is in a wrap, with lots of crunchy slaw and home-made tzatziki.

SERVES 3–4

FOR THE MEATBALLS
½ onion, finely diced
2 garlic cloves, grated or crushed
2½ tbsp coconut oil
500g lean lamb mince
1 free-range egg
1 tbsp fresh mint, chopped
1 tbsp fresh dill, chopped
Salt and black pepper

FOR THE TZATZIKI
480g Greek yogurt
½ cucumber, deseeded and diced
Juice of ½ lemon
2 garlic cloves, crushed
2 tbsp fresh mint, chopped
1 tbsp fresh dill, chopped
Salt and black pepper

TO SERVE
6–8 tortilla wraps
crunchy slaw

Preheat the oven to 180°C/350°F/gas mark 4.

In a saucepan, sauté the onion and garlic in half a tablespoon of the coconut oil over a medium heat until translucent. Let it cool and set aside.

Combine the mince, egg, herbs, and cooled onion and garlic mixture in a large mixing bowl. Add a pinch of salt and pepper and mix well. Using your hands make 15–20 small meatballs from the mixture.

Add the remaining coconut oil to a large frying pan and cook the meatballs on all sides for 5–10 minutes until brown. You may need to do this in batches depending on the size of the pan.

Place the meatballs on a large baking tray lined with greaseproof paper and bake for a further 8–10 minutes until cooked right through.

While the meatballs are cooking, combine the ingredients for the tzatziki in a bowl and allow it to chill in the fridge.

When the meatballs are cooked, serve with tortilla wraps, tzatziki and a crunchy slaw.

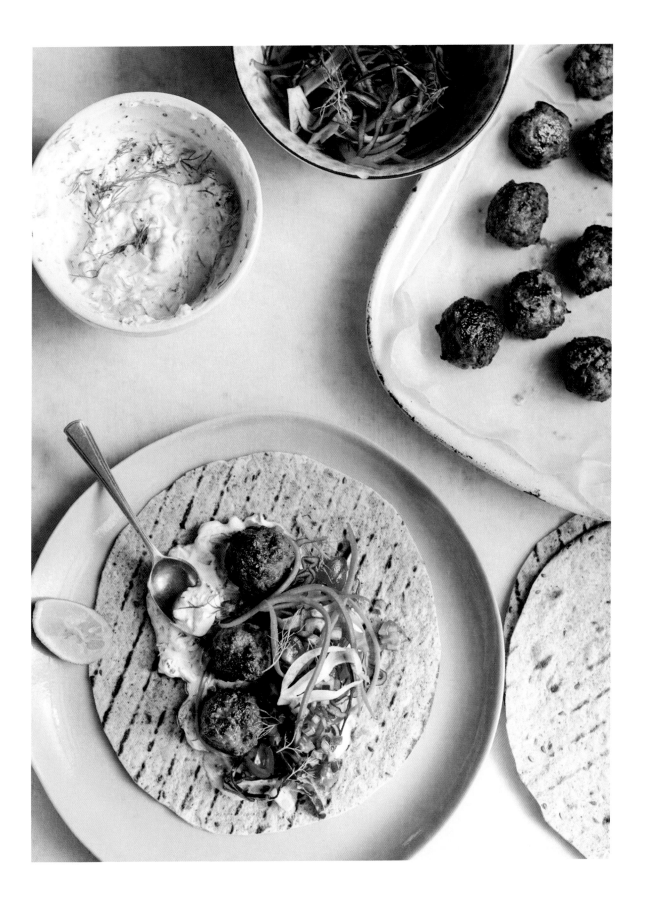

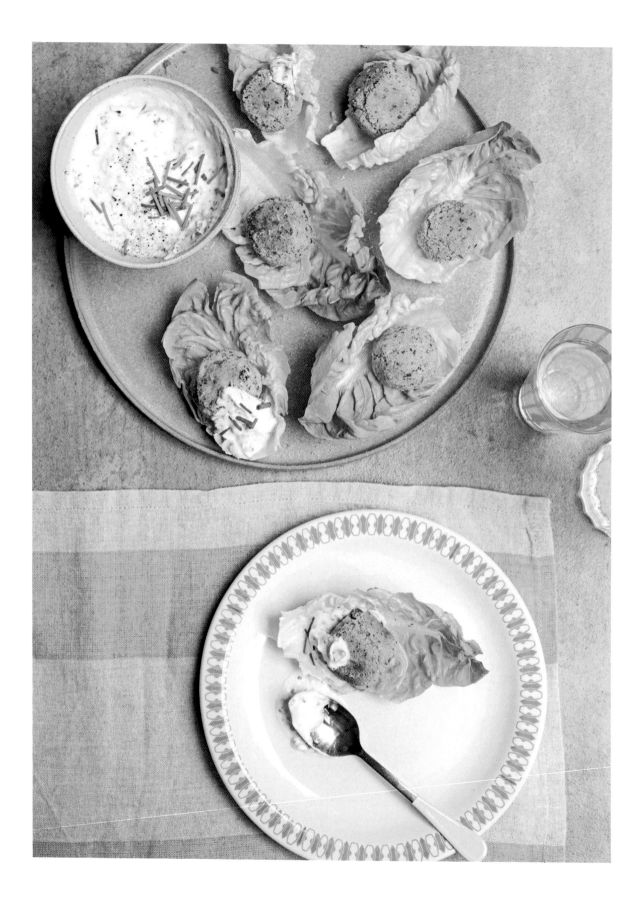

PEA + SPINACH FALAFEL WITH LEMON + GARLIC YOGURT DIP

I absolutely love falafel but it's so hard to find good falafel that isn't either totally dry or coated in breadcrumbs. I made this recipe for my first ever supper club and it had such amazing feedback! Everyone was asking for the recipe but I kept it under wraps until now. The mixture is quite wet and delicate, so in order to keep the inside moist and the outside crispy, make sure to coat the base of the pan in a layer of coconut oil, and carefully turn them only when required. Alternatively, you can cook these in the oven but I think they're best if they're at least sealed in the pan first.

SERVES 2–3

FOR THE FALAFEL
1 x 400g tin of chickpeas, rinsed and drained
30g garden peas, cooked
30g spinach
1½ tbsp tahini
Juice of ½ lemon
1 heaped tsp smoked paprika
1 tsp salt
2 tbsp coconut oil
Black pepper

FOR THE LEMON + GARLIC YOGURT DRESSING
150g Greek yogurt
1 tbsp lemon juice
1 garlic clove, crushed
2 tbsp chives, finely chopped
Salt and black pepper

TO SERVE
2 baby gem lettuce heads

Place the chickpeas and peas in a food processor and blend until you achieve a chunky paste.

Tear up the spinach and add it to the food processor.

Next add the tahini, lemon juice, paprika, salt and a sprinkle of pepper. Blend the mixture, stopping to scrape down the sides occasionally.

Blend until a sticky consistency is achieved: the mixture should come away from the sides of the food processor. If it's too dry and crumbly, gradually add some more tahini.

Shape the mixture into approximately 16 golf-ball sized rounds.

Put a large non-stick frying pan over a high heat and add the coconut oil – you should have enough to cover the base of the pan, add more as required.

Place the balls onto the hot pan and allow them to cook until golden and crispy on each side (beware of the oil spitting). Once they are golden on each side, reduce the heat to a low setting and allow the balls to cook right through for another 10 minutes. Remove from the heat and place on kitchen paper to soak up the excess coconut oil.

To make the dressing, combine all the ingredients in a bowl and season with salt and pepper to taste.

Serve in fresh lettuce boats with the lemon and garlic yogurt dressing on top.

QUINOA STUFFED SQUASH

This recipe comes from Emma, my beautiful big sister (see page 167). Emma is also a big healthy foodie, but unlike me, she is vegetarian. For Christmas last year we put our heads together to create this veggie alternative for a stuffed turkey. I love my Christmas turkey, but this recipe knocks every roast out of the park.

SERVES 4

1 butternut squash, cut in half lengthways and deseeded
350ml vegetable stock
75g quinoa, rinsed
1 tbsp walnut oil
1 small white onion, diced
2 garlic cloves, crushed
1 tsp rosemary
1 tbsp dried cranberries
1 tbsp dried apricots, roughly chopped
1 tbsp walnuts, chopped
1 tbsp parsley
2 tbsp fresh orange juice
Salt and black pepper

Twine (natural and undyed)

Preheat the oven to 180°C/350°F/gas mark 4.

Score the flesh of each butternut squash half with a sharp knife, then wrap each half in tinfoil and place them on the middle shelf of the oven for 30–40 minutes until the flesh becomes tender (you can test it with a butter knife – if it pierces the flesh easily then it's ready).

While the squash is cooking, prepare the quinoa. In a small saucepan with a lid, bring the stock to the boil and then add the quinoa. Allow the stock to come back up to the boil again. Reduce the heat, put on the lid and allow it to simmer for 20–25 minutes. Stir occasionally to ensure that the quinoa is cooking evenly and is not sticking to the bottom of the pan. The quinoa should be fully cooked once it is tender and all of the stock is being absorbed. You are aiming to have a wet, porridge-like consistency (rather than fluffy rice-like consistency – this is important to allow the stuffing to combine and hold).

In a small frying pan, gently heat the walnut oil and add the onion, garlic and rosemary. Add a little pinch of salt to help the onion sweat and cook the combined mixture until the onion becomes tender and turns slightly golden brown. Be careful not to burn the onion or the garlic.

In a large bowl, combine the cooked quinoa, and onion and garlic mixture using a wooden spoon or large spatula. Next add in the dried fruit, walnuts, parsley and orange juice, and mix well. Taste and season with salt and pepper – usually half a teaspoon of pepper and a pinch of salt is enough, as the stock and onion mixture will make the stuffing quite salty already. Set the stuffing mixture aside.

Remove the squash from the oven and allow it to cool. Once it is cool enough to handle, scoop out an approximately 1in groove in each half – be very careful not to scoop too close to the skin or the squash will not hold its form when you carve it for serving. Approximately 1 cup of butternut

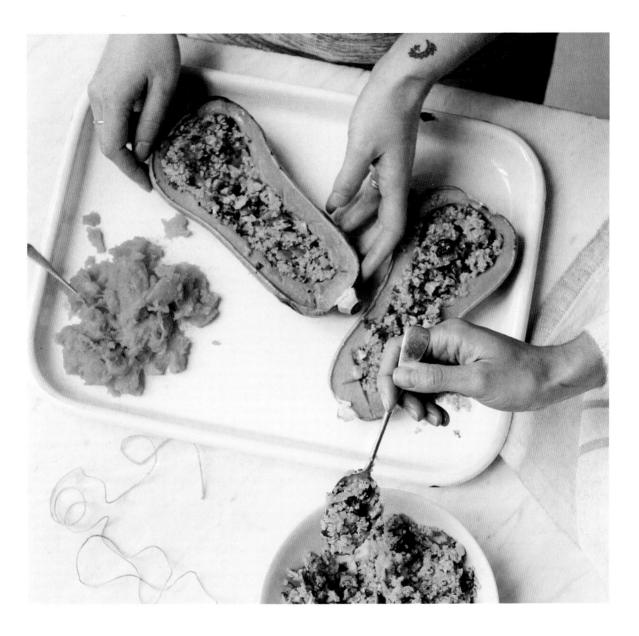

squash will be left over after scooping out the groove – you can serve it as a side or keep it in the fridge for lunch the next day.

Stuff each of the butternut squash halves with the stuffing mixture – really pack it in. Sandwich the 2 sides together and fasten them together with twine, tying it lengthways and crosswise. Wrap the squash in tinfoil and place it back in the oven for another 20–30 minutes.

Once cooked, remove it from the oven and carefully carve the squash into thick 2in slices to serve.

SWEET POTATO NACHOS + CHILLI

This is the ultimate Friday-night-in comfort food. As a self-confessed Mexican foodie, there is nothing I love more than a cocktail and a bowl of loaded Mexican nachos with the girls on a Friday night. Sadly for us, regular loaded nachos that you buy out are far from healthy despite containing lots of great ingredients like beef or chicken, avocado and tomatoes. So instead of a weekend takeaway, how about a weekend 'take-in'? I promise you once you try this out for yourself and see how easy it is to make, on top of how good it tastes, you won't be reaching for the local Mexican takeaway menu any more. This recipe is for beef chilli loaded nachos but you can swap the beef for chicken or a veggie option, such as black beans. I like to top my nachos with my home-made guacamole, salsa and a big dollop of thick Greek yogurt or Quark.

SERVES 4

FOR THE BEEF CHILLI
2 garlic cloves, grated
1 red onion, finely chopped
400–500g lean minced beef
1 red pepper, finely chopped
1 heaped tsp chilli powder
1 tsp smoked paprika
1 x 400g tin of kidney beans
1 x 400g tin of chopped tomatoes
280ml vegetable stock
Salt and black pepper

FOR THE SWEET POTATO NACHOS
2 large sweet potatoes, peeled and
    sliced into ¼in thick slices
1 tbsp melted coconut oil
1 tsp paprika
¼ tsp salt

SERVING SUGGESTIONS
Avocado, Greek yogurt, salsa,
mozzarella cheese

Preheat the oven to 180°C/350°F/gas mark 4. Toss the slices of sweet potato in the coconut oil, paprika and salt. Line 2 flat roasting trays with baking paper and arrange the potato slices in a single layer. Bake for 30–40 minutes, turning halfway to make sure they bake on both sides.

Place a large saucepan over a medium heat and sauté the garlic and onion in a large pan until soft. Add the mince and cook for 5–10 minutes until browned. Add the red pepper, chilli powder and paprika, and cook for 1 minute.

Drain the kidney beans and add them to the vegetables, along with the tomatoes. Add the stock to the chilli mixture. Bring everything to the boil and simmer for 20 minutes. Season with salt and pepper to taste.

Arrange the sweet potato slices on 1 large serving plate and spoon the chilli on top. Add whatever toppings you wish.

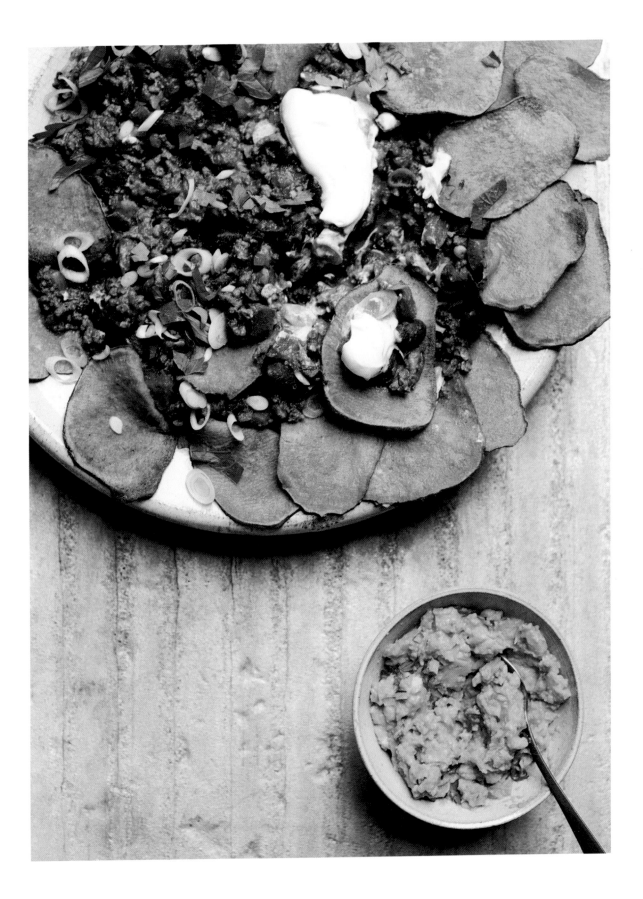

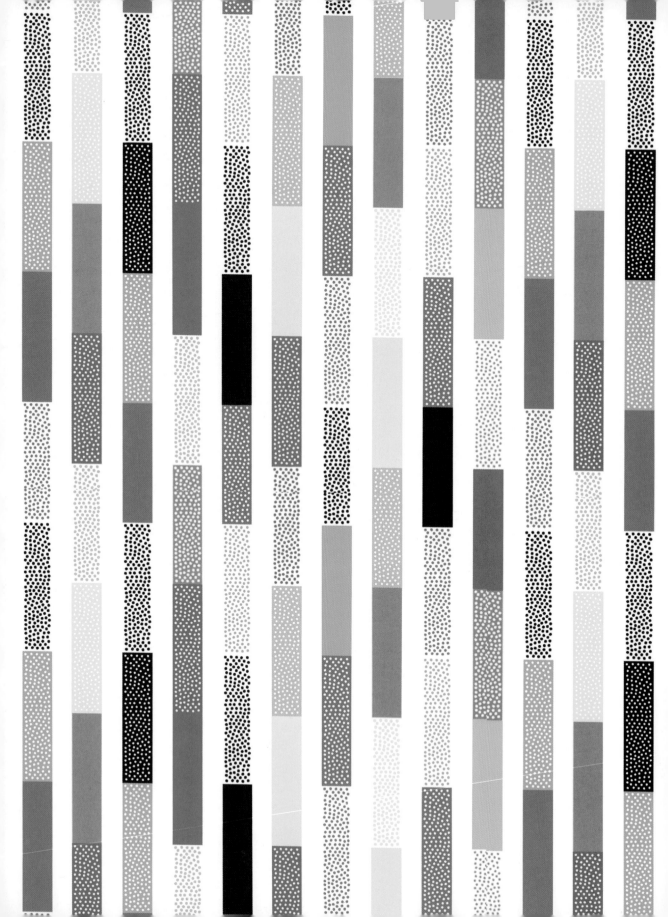

DESSERTS
+
SNACKS

*No matter how much
I eat, there's always
room for dessert.*

No matter how much I eat, there's always room for dessert.
It doesn't go to the stomach, it goes to the heart.

I love this slogan – it's so true! I've always had a sweet
tooth and I love to finish my evening meal with something
sweet – even if it's just a few squares of 85 per cent dark
chocolate. One of the reasons I advocate a balanced diet
is because a diet that doesn't allow flexibility can lead to
extremes of restrictive eating practices followed by periods
of binges – and then the feelings of guilt that follow.

Although we need to eat well for our health and our body,
we also need to eat for our soul – and that includes dessert!
The recipes in this section are designed to nourish both the
body and the soul – not only are they delicious, but they're
made from wholesome ingredients with minimal added
sugar. If you're like me and get peckish around 11 a.m.,
knock up a batch of no-bake cinnamon oatmeal energy balls
(page 212) or chocolate coconut protein balls (page 213) to
take to work.

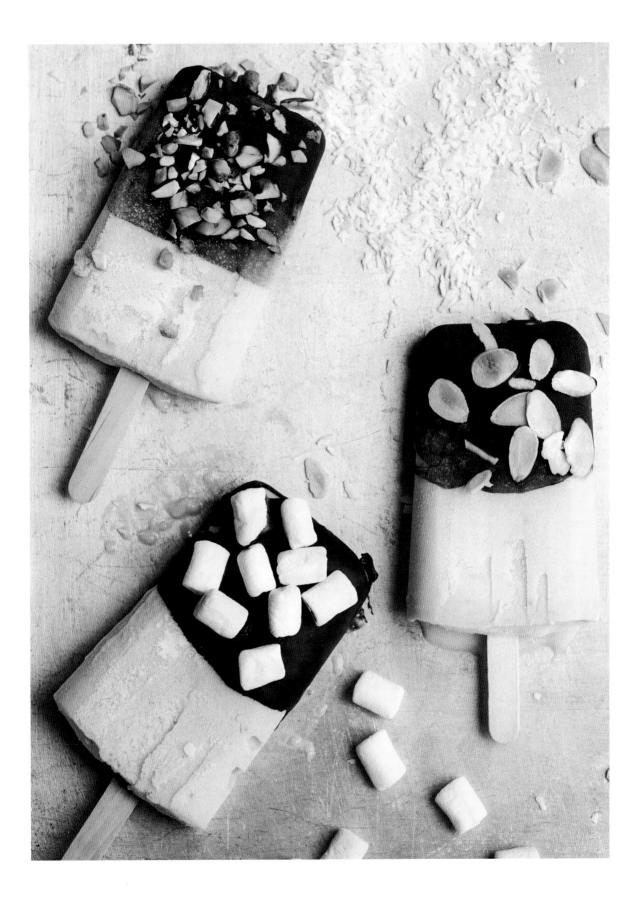

OLD-FASHIONED OATMEAL, CINNAMON + RAISIN COOKIES

My favourite cookie flavour has always been oatmeal, cinnamon and raisin. I just don't tire of them, especially the amazing smell they leave in the kitchen after I've baked a fresh batch. I've tried and tested lots of different ways to 'healthify' the classic cookie, which is packed full of refined sugar, and I've finally perfected my recipe.

MAKES 12–14 COOKIES

100g fine-cut or instant porridge oats
100g plain gluten-free flour (I use Dove's), sifted*
1 tsp baking powder**
2 tsp ground cinnamon
¼ tsp salt
1 tbsp coconut oil
1 heaped tbsp smooth almond butter
120ml honey or agave nectar
1 tsp vanilla extract
1 free-range egg
40g raisins

The gluten-free flour can be substituted for plain flour.

** *Use gluten-free if required.*

Whisk together the oats, flour, baking powder, cinnamon and salt in a large mixing bowl.

Place the coconut oil and almond butter in a microwaveable bowl and microwave for 20 seconds until the coconut oil melts. Stir in the honey or agave nectar and the vanilla extract, and mix until combined.

Pour the coconut oil mixture over the dry ingredients, add the egg and stir well. Fold in the raisins.

Cover and refrigerate the cookie dough for 20–30 minutes to allow the mixture to stiffen.

Preheat the oven to 180°C/350°F/gas mark 4 and line 2 flat baking trays with greaseproof paper.

Using a tablespoon, scoop out 12–14 portions of the cookie dough onto the trays. Flatten down each scoop slightly. Bake for 10 minutes and let them cool on the trays for 10 minutes before transferring them to a wire rack.

TIP: *For a nut-free version, the almond butter can be substituted for coconut oil or butter.*

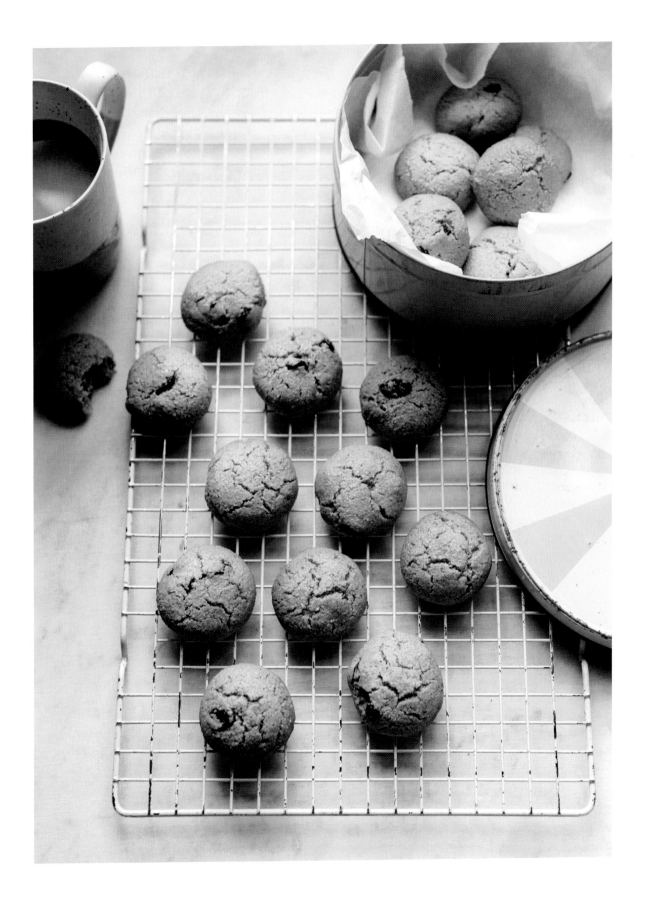

CHOCOLATE SWEET POTATO PUDDING

I love using sweet potato in both sweet and savoury dishes. Although this dish may sound a little bit too outlandish for some, please don't knock it until you try it. It's one of my favourite comfort snacks to munch on while watching a movie. It requires only a handful of ingredients and it doesn't take long to make either. To top it off, it's low in refined sugar and packed full of vitamins, minerals and fibre.

SERVES 2

1 large sweet potato, peeled and cut into chunks
1 tbsp coconut oil, melted
1 tsp cinnamon
4 medjool dates, pitted
1 tbsp honey or agave nectar
1 tbsp smooth peanut butter or almond butter
3 tbsp cacao powder or cocoa powder
40g dark chocolate, chopped (optional)

Preheat the oven to 180°C/350°F/gas mark 4. Place the sweet potato on a lined baking tray and toss in the melted coconut oil and cinnamon. Bake for 30–35 minutes until soft. Allow to cool for at least 1–2 hours.

Soak the dates in boiling water for 10–20 minutes. Take the cooled sweet potato and process it in a food processor until smooth. You may need to stop several times to scrape down the sides.

Drain the dates and discard the water. Add the dates, honey or agave nectar, nut butter and cacao to the sweet potato and blend until smooth and creamy.

Fold in the dark chocolate and store in the fridge until ready to serve.

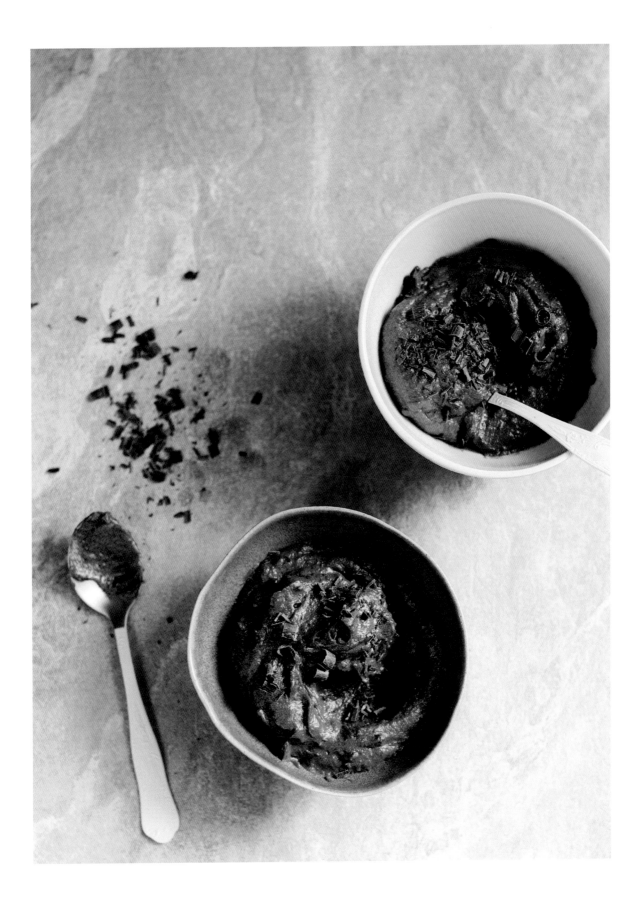

CHOCOLATE SWIRL BANANA BREAD

Banana bread is the perfect (and tastiest) solution for using up over-ripe bananas. Unlike traditional banana bread recipes that call for refined white flour and white sugar, this recipe is made with coconut flour and is naturally sweetened with honey. I've also swapped the margarine for coconut oil which is full of healthy fats.

You could make this banana bread even healthier by omitting the chocolate – but this I wouldn't recommend, because a little bit of chocolate is good for the soul.

MAKES 10–12 SLICES

120g coconut flour
1 tsp cinnamon
½ tsp baking powder*
½ tsp bicarbonate of soda
¼ tsp salt
6 free-range eggs
80g honey
75g coconut oil, melted
   and cooled, plus extra to grease
120ml almond milk
1 tsp vanilla extract
3 ripe bananas, mashed
75g 85 per cent dark chocolate,
   chopped
½ banana, sliced, to top

* Use gluten-free if required.

Preheat the oven to 180°C/350°F/gas mark 4. Prepare a large loaf pan (silicone works best) by greasing the sides with a little coconut oil.

In a large mixing bowl, mix the coconut flour, cinnamon, baking powder, bicarbonate of soda and salt. In another large bowl, beat the eggs. Add the honey, coconut oil, almond milk and vanilla extract to the eggs, and whisk very well to combine.

Pour the dry ingredients into the bowl of wet ingredients, and whisk very well until combined. Mix in the mashed banana.

Melt the dark chocolate in the microwave for 60–90 seconds, stirring every 30 seconds. Fold the dark chocolate into the banana bread mixture very gently without over-mixing so the 2 mixtures form a marbled effect.

Pour the batter into the prepared loaf pan and add the sliced banana on top. Bake uncovered for 45 minutes, then cover with a sheet of tinfoil and bake for another 15 minutes or until a toothpick inserted into the centre comes out clean. The cake will be quite moist in texture but should not be wet.

Cool in the pan for about 20 minutes. Remove the loaf from the pan and allow it to cool completely on a wire rack for about an hour, before slicing.

PS... You can store the bread in the fridge for 3–5 days, or in the freezer in a ziplock bag for up to 3 months.

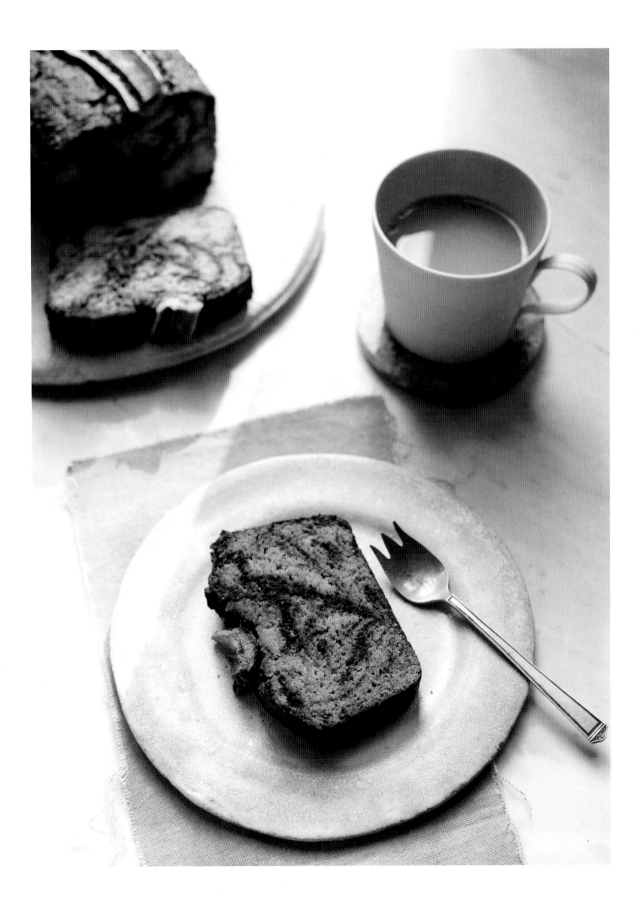

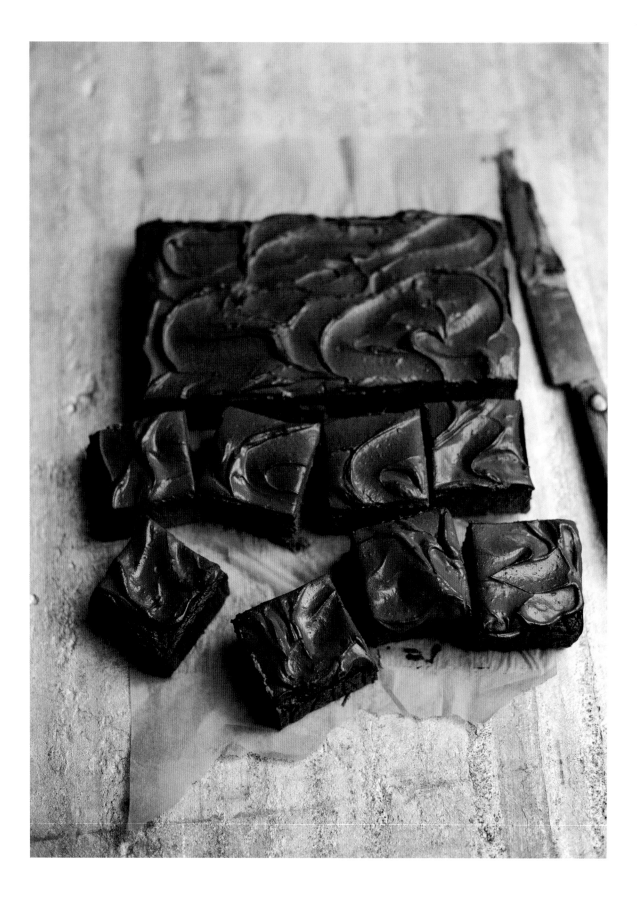

CHOCOLATE ORANGE SWEET POTATO BROWNIES

One of my favourite recipes is sweet potato protein brownies. They are so quick and easy to make that I often knock them up on a Sunday evening to bring as a snack to work. I've revamped my old recipe with this chocolate orange version and added a delicious, creamy icing. At 100kcal a piece, these goodies are not to be passed up.

MAKES 16

Coconut oil, to grease
500g sweet potato, peeled and chopped
2 tbsp coconut sugar*
60g ground almonds
60g chocolate whey protein powder**
25g cacao or cocoa powder, sifted
Zest and juice of 1 large orange
1 tsp baking powder***
3 free-range egg whites

FOR THE ICING
55g dark chocolate chips
1 tbsp cacao or cocoa powder, sifted
120g Greek yogurt

May be substituted for an alternative sugar or powdered sweetener.

**Can be substituted for vegan protein powder or if you wish to omit the protein completely, try substituting it with cocoa powder or skimmed milk powder.*

***Use gluten-free if required.*

Preheat the oven to 180°C/350°F/gas mark 4. Prepare an 8in x 8in baking tin by greasing the sides and base with coconut oil.

Boil the sweet potato in a saucepan of water for 10–15 minutes until soft. Drain the excess water, place the sweet potato in a bowl and mash using a potato masher or a hand blender.

In a large mixing bowl, add the coconut sugar, ground almonds, protein powder, cacao, orange zest and baking powder. Stir.

Add the egg whites and 2 tablespoons of the juice from the orange to the dry mixture, and set the remaining juice aside for the icing. Finally add the mashed potato to the mixture and stir until no lumps remain.

Pour the brownie batter into the baking tin and bake for 30–35 minutes, or until a toothpick comes out clean.

Allow the brownies to cool for 30 minutes before removing them from the tin and placing them on a wire-rack for another 2–3 hours. The brownies must be completely cool before icing.

To make the icing, melt the dark chocolate in a microwave for a minute or 2, stopping every 30 seconds to stir, ensuring it doesn't burn. Add 2 tablespoons of the leftover orange juice and stir well.

Add the cacao powder and Greek yogurt to the melted chocolate and stir well until smooth.

Spread the icing on top of the brownie and allow it to chill in the fridge for 30 minutes before slicing it into 16 squares.

NOT-SO-BORING PEACH + STRAWBERRY CRUMBLE

Most Sundays, my mum would make apple crumble for dessert, using the apples from the tree in our orchard. As kids we would take turns to help her and it wasn't long before we were making it on our own. There's an old family story (which my family still won't let me live down) where I asked my mum what was for dessert and cheekily followed it by saying 'boring aul apple crumble again, is it?' Now everyone in my family refers to apple crumble as 'boring aul apple crumble'.

So I've revamped the crumble that my mother taught me to make with peaches and strawberries and substituted the butter in the crumble with some extra-virgin coconut oil.

SERVES 6

FOR THE CRUMBLE
100g oats
45g ground almonds
45g flaked almonds
2 tbsp coconut sugar*
1 tsp cinnamon
50g coconut oil, unmelted

FOR THE FILLING
4 peaches, stoned and sliced
150g strawberries, washed and
  halved
Juice of ½ lemon
1 tbsp coconut sugar*
1 tsp cinnamon

TO SERVE
1 x 500g tub of Greek yogurt

May be substituted for brown sugar, agave nectar or honey.

Preheat the oven to 180°C/350°F/gas mark 4. Toss all the ingredients for the filling together and place the mixture in a deep pie dish.

In a mixing bowl, combine the oats, ground almonds, flaked almonds, coconut sugar and cinnamon.

Next add the coconut oil, in several pieces at a time and, using your hands, work it into the mixture. Break up the larger lumps with the tips of your fingers until you have a fine crumble mixture. Spread the crumble mixture on top of the fruit, ensuring it's entirely covered. Pat down with the palm of your hand or a wooden spoon.

Bake for 30–35 minutes, until the crumble is golden. Cover with a sheet of tinfoil if the crumble is browning too quickly and cook for another 10 minutes.

Remove from the oven and allow to cool for 10 minutes before serving with fresh Greek yogurt.

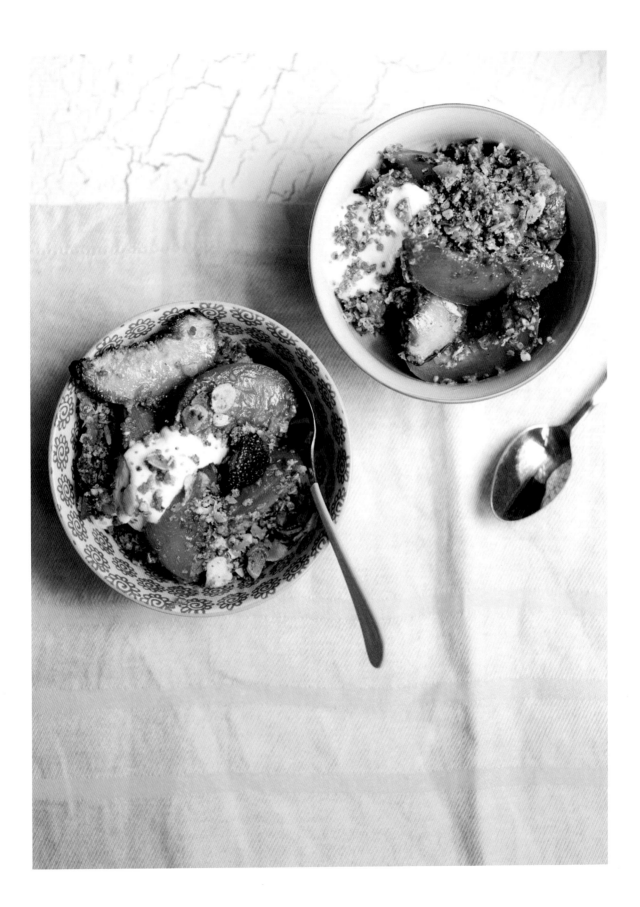

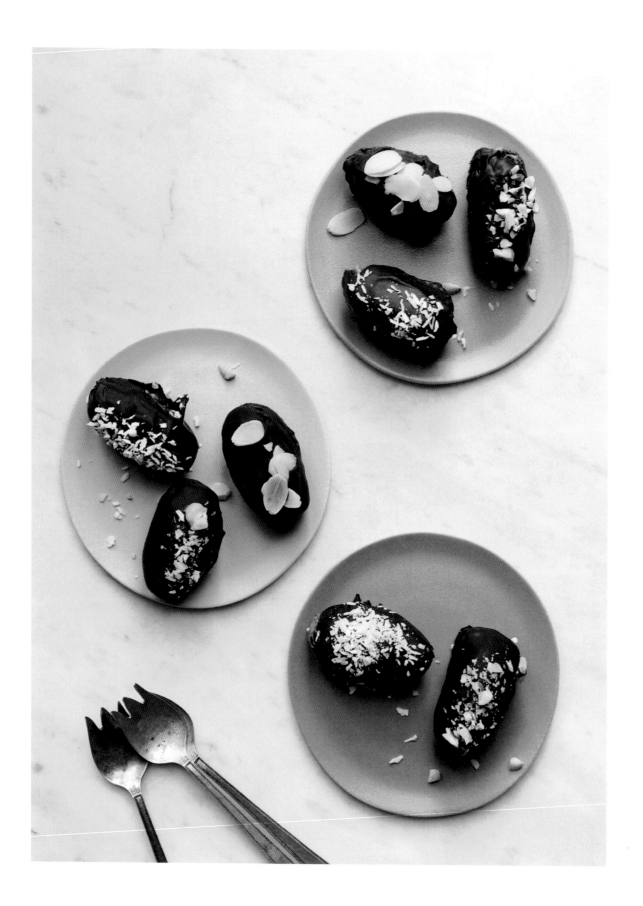

CHOCOLATE-COATED PEANUT BUTTER STUFFED DATES

At Christmas, my favourite sport is wrestling for the hard toffees in the box of chocolates. However, these truffles are a lot healthier than those you find at the bottom of a sweet tin. As you can probably guess from the name, these sweets have only three ingredients: dates, peanut butter and dark chocolate. The toppings are optional, but I recommend including them, particularly the desiccated coconut. However, although these little treats are 100 per cent natural, they still count as a treat and you need to try to stick to one or two pieces per serving.

12 SERVINGS

12 medjool dates
6 tsp peanut butter
40g 85 per cent dark chocolate, melted

OPTIONAL TOPPINGS
Crushed hazelnuts, flaked almonds, desiccated coconut

Slice the dates lengthways and remove the pits. Spoon half a teaspoon of peanut butter inside each date.

Place the dates on a flat tray lined with baking parchment and freeze them for 2–3 hours.

Melt the chocolate in the microwave in bursts of 30 seconds, ensuring it doesn't burn.

Roll the frozen dates in the melted chocolate. If using additional toppings, roll the chocolate-covered dates in the topping and place them back on the baking parchment.

Once you've finished coating each date, place them in the fridge or back in the freezer. Store in the fridge for a softer filling or in the freezer for a harder toffee-like filling.

BANANA 'NICE CREAM' POPSICLES

Dairy-free, vegan, low-calorie and all-natural ice cream anyone? If you haven't tried making ice cream with frozen bananas yet, you haven't lived. This genius idea is the best substitute for ice cream – it's just as creamy and just as delicious. Simply whizz the frozen bananas up in a blender until creamy, scoop the bananas into a bowl and eat the 'ice cream' as it is or take it to a whole other level and make popsicles with the mixture. This also makes a great sweet alternative for kids. Get them involved in the process by choosing their favourite toppings to dip the popsicles in.

MAKES 6 POPSICLES

3 bananas, frozen
120ml almond milk
40g dark chocolate
½ tbsp coconut oil

TOPPINGS
Chopped nuts, flaked almonds, mini marshmallows, desiccated coconut

Combine the bananas and almond milk in a blender. Blend until smooth, stopping the food processor or blender every so often to scrape the sides and push the banana back towards the middle.

Spoon the creamy banana mixture into popsicle moulds and freeze for 5–6 hours. Remove them from the freezer 10–15 minutes before topping to allow easy removal from the moulds.

To make the chocolate topping, microwave the chocolate in a small bowl for 30–60 seconds, stirring once or twice. Add the coconut oil and microwave for another 10 seconds. Stir the melted chocolate and coconut oil mixture together.

Sprinkle the toppings you wish to use on a plate. Prepare a baking tray with baking parchment. Remove the banana pops from the freezer and carefully take them out of their moulds. Dip the pops into the chocolate or drizzle it on top, and then dip them into the toppings. Place the pops on the baking tray and place the baking tray in the freezer until the chocolate shell is completely set. These can be stored in the freezer for several days.

VARIATIONS
- **CHOCOLATE BANANA ICE CREAM**
  Add 1–2 tablespoons of cacao or cocoa powder to the blended mixture.
- **PEANUT BANANA ICE CREAM**
  Add 2 tablespoons of smooth peanut butter, or peanut flour, to the blended mixture.
- **RASPBERRY BANANA ICE CREAM**
  Add a handful of frozen raspberries to the blended mixture.

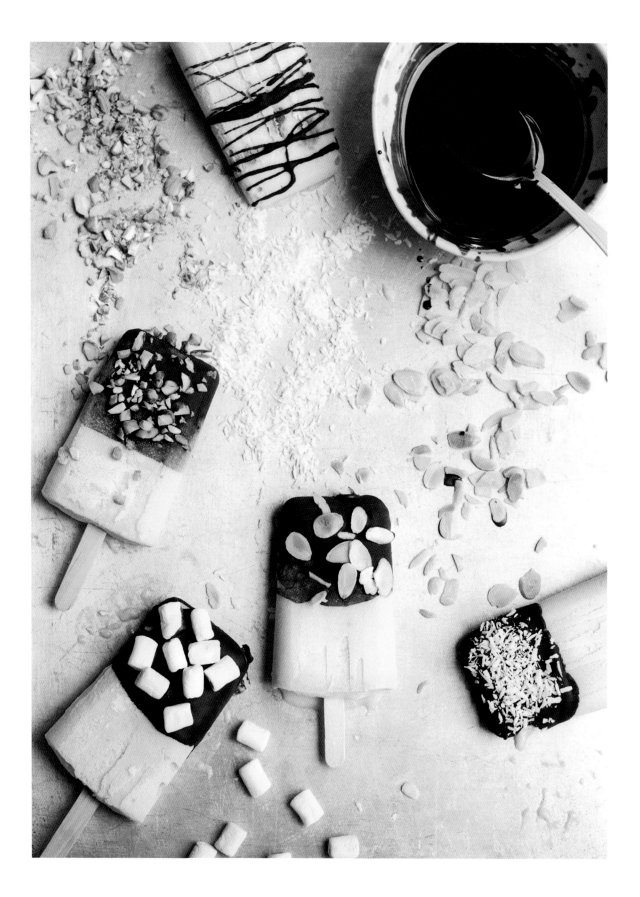

NO-BAKE CINNAMON OATMEAL ENERGY BALLS

These energy bites are so addictive and quite literally packed full of good stuff. This protein ball recipe is actually free of protein supplements – all of the protein comes from the peanut butter, chia seeds and oats.

MAKES 12–14

100g oats
1 tbsp chia
2 tsp cinnamon
40g raisins
1 tbsp coconut oil, melted
50g honey or agave nectar
50g peanut butter

Place the oats, chia, cinnamon and raisins in a large mixing bowl and mix together.

Combine the coconut oil, honey or agave nectar and peanut butter in a separate bowl.

Pour the wet mixture into the dry mixture to form a sticky dough that comes away from the sides of the bowl. If it is too dry, add a little more honey or agave nectar; alternatively, if it is too sticky add a little more oats.

Separate the mixture into approximately 12–14 tablespoon-sized balls.

Place them in the fridge on a baking tray to firm up for 30 minutes before serving.

CHOCOLATE COCONUT PROTEIN BALLS

These protein-packed, portable bites are the perfect snack to pop in your lunchbox. They can be whipped up in 5 minutes, require no baking, and last in the fridge for 3–5 days or in the freezer for up to 3 months in an airtight container.

MAKES 12

75g cashews
30g dessicated coconut
2 tbsp coconut flour
25g protein powder
1 tbsp cocoa powder
2½ tbsp coconut oil, melted
2 tbsp honey or agave nectar

In a food processor, blend the cashew nuts, coconut, coconut flour, protein powder and cocoa powder into a crumb-like consistency.

Next add the coconut oil and honey or agave nectar. Blend until well combined and the mix resembles a dough – add a splash of water if it is too dry or extra coconut flour if it is too wet.

Form the mixture into approximately 12 golf-ball sized balls.

Place in the fridge on a baking tray to set and store in an airtight container.

ONE-MINUTE CHOCOLATE PROTEIN BROWNIE

This is my go-to-recipe when I fancy something sweet after dinner. Made with just five ingredients, in under five minutes, this brownie recipe will change your life. To add to its appeal, it is super-low in sugar, high in protein and really low-calorie. So on this occasion, don't be afraid to have your cake and eat it.

SERVES 1

Coconut oil, to grease
2 tbsp chocolate whey protein
1 tbsp coconut flour
½ tsp baking powder*
1 free-range egg white
70ml milk

* Use gluten-free if required

Grease a small serving bowl or mug with a little bit of coconut oil.

In a mixing bowl, combine the dry ingredients. In a separate bowl, whisk the egg white with the milk, pour the mixture into the dry mixture and mix until fully incorporated.

Microwave the mixture for 60 seconds (watching carefully that it doesn't spill over the sides), stop and microwave for another 15–30 seconds until the top is firm.

Turn over onto a plate and serve.

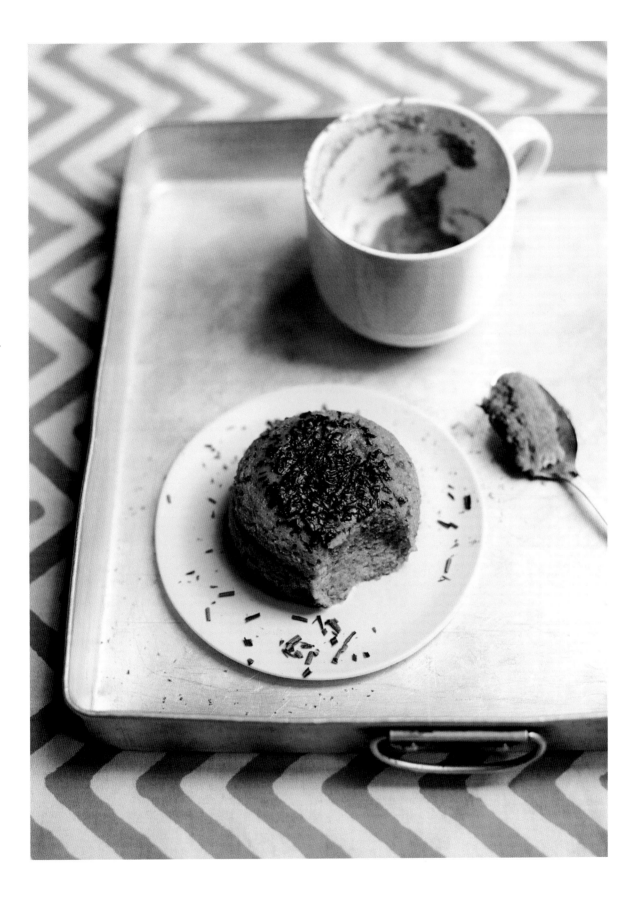

PROTEIN SOFT SERVE

It may sound bizarre but it tastes like whipped ice cream and once you try it, you won't be able to stop making it. It's made from three basic ingredients: protein powder, xanthan gum and milk. The xanthan gum is a type of fibre which acts as a thickening agent and gives it an incredible marshmallowy texture. With less than 150kcal per serving and over 20g of protein, it's the perfect evening treat.

SERVES 1

25g vanilla protein powder
(1 scoop)
Handful of ice cubes
½ tsp xanthan gum
250ml unsweetened almond
milk

Place all the ingredients into a blender or food processor and blend for 1–2 minutes until thick and creamy.

VARIATIONS
- Different flavours of protein powder
- Frozen berries, pineapple, apple or banana
- Cocoa powder

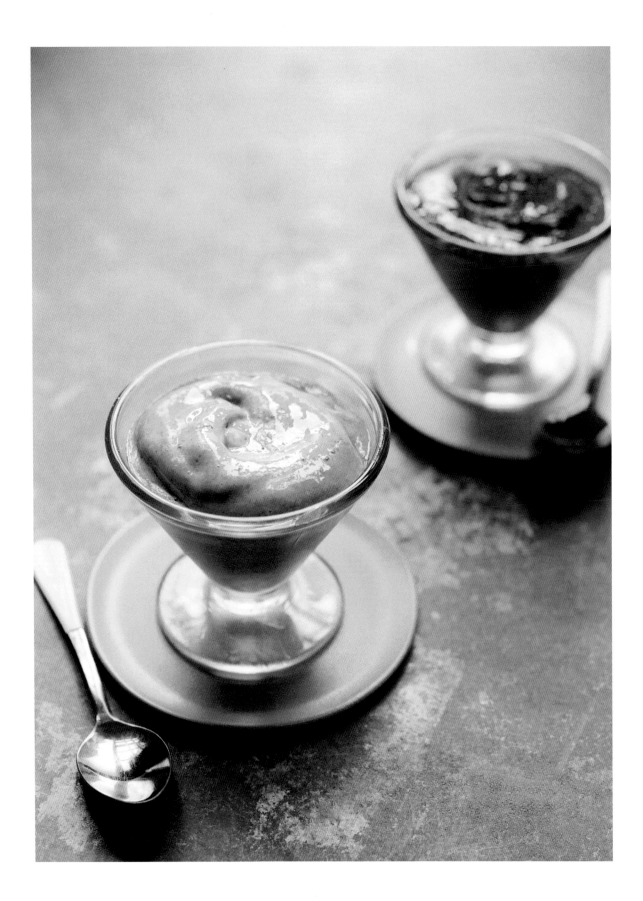

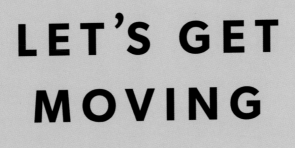

'Movement is medicine for changing a person's physical, emotional, and mental state.' ANONYMOUS

We all exercise for different reasons – to lose weight, to gain muscle, to train for a marathon, or because our doctor told us to. Personally, I don't put those reasons at the top of my list. Now don't get me wrong, I love the health improvements and changes in my body that come from lifting weights, but when I reflected on my reasons for training, I realised that the benefits strength training offers me mentally far outweighs the physical ones.

As a child, I was very athletic, with a huge passion for sports. I grew up playing all sorts of sports: soccer, Gaelic football, horseriding, gymnastics, tennis, badminton, golf, basketball, hockey and athletics . . . basically, if there was a team, I wanted to be on it. If there was a competition, I wanted to compete. My dad was massively into sports himself and after he retired, he would attend all of my games and competitions. After he died, my interest in sport slowly dwindled away. The rest of my family didn't share the same passion that my dad and I had, and I guess not having someone to sit and watch the Man United match or kick a football around the garden with, made me shy away from sports all together.

During the period when I was severely underweight, I found it difficult to do any form of exercise without becoming exhausted. I spent most of my time at home at my desk wrapped up in layers of clothing to keep warm, even on the hottest days of the year. When I started to see the dietician, she suggested that I started incorporating some gentle exercise. Initially, I was hesitant and for a good reason: my BMI was less than 15, my health was unstable and I was trying to gain weight, not lose it. However, what I failed to understand initially was that exercise in this context was not for weight loss but for improvements in physical and mental strength. I had no muscle mass on my body so my strength was similar to that of a ninety-year-old woman and my exercise tolerance would allow me to walk only short distances before I needed to rest.

I started with walks in the evening, once or twice a week, down to our local village and back. I would take my iPod and our shih-tzu dog, Millie, and escape from everything going on in my life for a brief thirty minutes. I also enrolled on an eight-week yoga course with my mum, which in all honesty didn't offer me much in the way of physical benefits but did wonders for my mind. The deep breathing techniques and meditation allowed me to find peace in a world that had been consumed by chaos and quieten my thoughts for a brief moment. After months of not finding joy in anything, I started to feel happier and more relaxed after my weekly yoga sessions and evening walks. I stopped fearing that exercise would impede the speed of my recovery and began to understand how important it was in my recovery process – both for my mind and my body.

The story changed quite a bit when I went to university and first discovered weight training. This time I was calling upon exercise to help me lose the weight I had gained, to build muscle and to improve my low self-esteem.

I stepped into my university gym with no experience and no idea what I was doing. The only time I had ever been to a gym before was to use the cardio machines and back then my idea of a successful workout was completely knackering myself on the treadmill for sixty minutes.

Before I started lifting weights, I spent weeks reading articles and watching YouTube videos before taking the plunge. 'Reps', 'sets', 'barbells' and 'kettlebells' were a whole new vocabulary for me.

I couldn't afford a personal trainer, but I could afford a student membership so I designed the most basic eight-week full body plan and decided to teach and train myself. This could have gone horribly wrong and to say I was like a sheep without a shepherd wandering around the gym would be a bit of an understatement! I would drive the instructors on the gym floor crazy by constantly asking them how to use the different machines or if my technique was correct. At first I felt embarrassed about how clueless I must have looked shouldering in next to all the big, burly men, curling my two-kilo dumb-bells. The funny thing is the men in the gym were totally supportive and took me under their wing, teaching me the right technique, and pushing me to lift heavier weights week-on-week.

I shifted my focus from counting calories burned on the treadmill to the strength increases I was making. Despite long days studying in the library or shadowing on the wards, I would still be itching to make it to the gym. It soon became my sanctuary, a place where I could escape from the stresses in my life and challenge myself physically, not mentally, for a change.

I've always pushed myself academically throughout my life, at school and then at university, but it wasn't until I challenged my body physically that I discovered my true inner strength. I think the biggest lesson I learnt was that failure is not final. I changed my way of thinking and approached failure as an opportunity for progress, not the opportunity to quit. I truly believe that it has shaped me into a more resilient, independent and fearless person.

Exercising to build muscle or lose weight is great if your goal is purely physical, but pushing through a hard workout does a lot more than strengthen your body – it strengthens your mind. Every session isn't about absolutely destroying yourself, but about taking yourself out of your comfort zone and having to dig deep to stand up to new challenges – that is when you truly become a stronger person. Sure, you can 'get it done' or beat the others, but if you aren't challenging yourself every conditioning session, you aren't discovering what you are truly capable of.

CARDIOVASCULAR vs STRENGTH TRAINING

Strength training, sometimes called resistance training, is a form of exercise that involves using your muscles to contract against a weight or force. The resistance used can be anything from dumb-bells, barbells, kettlebells, resistance bands, or simply your own body weight. The muscle gradually changes over time by increasing in strength and size.

To 'strength train' implies training with the purpose of getting stronger, but that's not the only benefit it offers you! Strength training makes you leaner by increasing your muscle mass and reducing your body fat. Basically, when people talk about being 'toned', this is what they mean. Muscles themselves do not 'firm up' or 'tone', but we can appear more 'toned' overall by training our muscles to have more definition and shape, and losing body fat.

'Cardio' is short for cardiovascular, which refers to the heart, lungs and blood vessels. There are lots of different forms of cardiovascular training but we can broadly categorise them into aerobic and anaerobic. The defining feature between the two forms of exercise is oxygen – aerobic means 'with oxygen' and anaerobic means 'without oxygen'.

Aerobic exercise uses oxygen to break down carbohydrate and fats for energy. This is a very efficient process of producing energy, but you can't work at maximum intensity. So you couldn't sprint for thirty minutes at maximum speed, but you could run for that length of time. Aerobic exercise is usually a form of low-intensity steady state cardio (LISS), such as running or cycling – unless you're sprinting or working at your max heart rate of course!

Anaerobic exercise involves shorter periods of higher-intensity exercise, like sprints or circuit training. Your body's demand for oxygen exceeds the oxygen supply available, and so energy is produced without oxygen via a different pathway. This is less efficient but it allows us to produce short bursts of energy rapidly – think of a box jump or a 100m sprint. Since the body can't work at this intensity for long periods of time, these sessions tend to be shorter and broken up into intervals with rest periods.

High-intensity interval training (HIIT) is a training method that uses the anaerobic energy system. HIIT involves alternate periods of pushing your body to its limit, i.e. high-intensity, with periods of rest or lower-intensity exercise, such as walking. HIIT can be done purely using your own body weight or you can mix it up with kettlebells, sandbags, dumb-bells, sledges, logs . . . basically anything to add to the intensity!

Both forms of training are effective and have been shown to improve cardiovascular health, blood pressure, cholesterol levels, insulin sensitivity and fat loss. There is a lot of debate as to which one is more effective but in terms of fat loss and muscle retention, research shows that HIIT appears to come out on top. In reality, these processes never work in isolation and our bodies tend to use both aerobic and anaerobic metabolism in any given training session.

Now this is not to say that low-intensity steady state (LISS) cardio does not have its advantages too. Compared to HIIT, it puts less stress and strain on the body which reduces the likelihood of injury. Those with orthopaedic problems, such as osteoarthritis, should opt for non-weight bearing, lower-intensity exercises, such as swimming and cycling. Many people prefer LISS cardio for relaxation purposes and there's nothing wrong with that.

However, if you're a busy individual – as many of us are these days – you definitely get more bang for your buck, in terms of efficiency, with HIIT. I'm a huge fan of training this way because although it is much more intense than other forms of exercise, it's much less time-consuming: I can squeeze a solid twenty-minute session into my schedule at any time. It's also really versatile, which keeps things interesting. You can change the exercises, the training protocol and the equipment you use, so each workout is completely different to the previous one. HIIT training is adaptable to any environment so you don't need a gym or any equipment to do it – you can do it in the park, at home, in a hotel or a gym! Another reason I'm a fan of HIIT is simply because I L-O-V-E it! I find it really hard to enjoy sixty minutes of steady-state cardio on the treadmill or rower – my mind tends to wander and my motivation lags towards the end. With HIIT, I'm changing from one exercise to the next or racing against the clock, so my motivation stays high and even increases throughout the workout.

In terms of my own training, it tends to be a bit sporadic! As a busy junior doctor, I can't always predict how my day is going to run. There are weeks I fit in three or four sessions at the gym and weeks when I won't make it there at all. This is why HIIT is a really important part of my training. On a perfect week, I like to do two sessions of my own strength-training programme, which involves lifting weights and doing compound exercises like squats and dead lifts, and then doing two additional HIIT sessions inside or outside of the gym. If my training does have to take a back seat for any reason, I don't stress about it but I make sure that I stay on top of my nutrition. Getting in enough protein, the right fats and wholesome carbohydrates means that I'm doing the very best I can to maintain my physical condition. If I stopped training and ate a diet full of junk food, my body would drastically change and I would set myself back in terms of health and physical conditioning. Taking a few days off and eating well gives my body the opportunity to rest and grow until I can get back into training.

YOU CAN'T OUT-TRAIN A BAD DIET

Exercise alone won't change your physique and an hour at the gym does not earn you a brownie! It's funny how often we justify our bad food choices because 'I worked out today'. Despite the calories-in/calories-out principle, you cannot out-train a bad diet. First of all, you shouldn't feel like you need to punish yourself at the gym for having the odd treat every once in a while and secondly, exercise really doesn't burn as many calories as people assume it does, so a single workout – even an intense one – won't come close to cancelling out a big binge. If weight loss is your goal, you have to stay on track and avoid going on weekend or late-night binges, otherwise you'll be fighting and losing an uphill battle. The same goes for your diet – improving your diet will result in some weight loss, but your body won't necessarily look strong and lean if you aren't regularly working those muscles.

PICK 'n' MIX HIIT WORKOUT

The best kind of training programme is one tailored to you that involves all the forms of training discussed earlier: weight training and aerobic and anaerobic cardio. As it is impossible for me to design a unique, tailored programme for each person who buys the book, I've come up with a way of making it personal to you.

I've designed a pick 'n' mix table of exercises which are broken down into four categories: A, B, C and D. Each category has a list of exercises that you can choose from to design your own HIIT circuit. This way you have the power to train what you want to train and you won't get bored doing the same old circuits week on week! There will be some exercises that you feel capable of doing and those that you may feel are too advanced for your level of fitness. The good news is that with your own HIIT workout, you can choose the exercises that you know are well within your abilities, and then build up to more difficult ones as you progress.

There are six different training protocols that you can slot the exercises into, giving you more autonomy and greater choice when it comes to your training and also offering you different options depending on how much time you have to train. Try to change which protocol you use each time to challenge yourself and keep things interesting.

To see results I recommend that you do three of these circuits a week, with an optional day of doing your own lower-intensity exercise, such as walking, running, cycling or swimming. If you're using this programme as part of your own strength training regime then use it once or twice a week, depending on how often you train, ensuring that you give yourself at least one full day off from any form of exercise to rest!

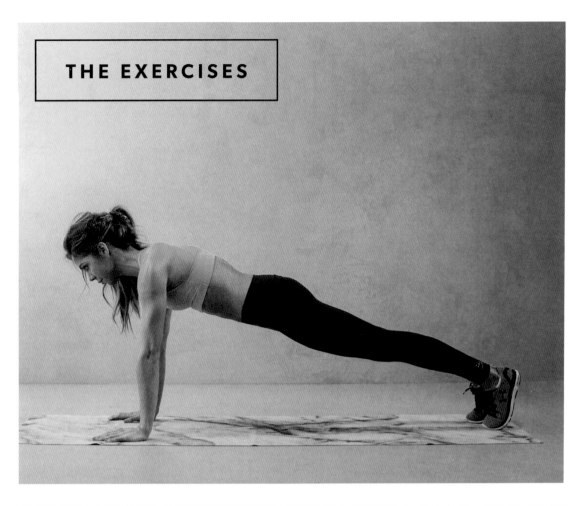

THE EXERCISES

A	B	C	D
Push-up	Side lunge	Ab crunches	Burpee
Tricep dip	Forward lunge	Flutter kick	Tuck jump
Plank to push-up	Bulgarian split squat	V-up	Jump lunge
Push-up with rotation	Squat	Mountain climber	Jump squat

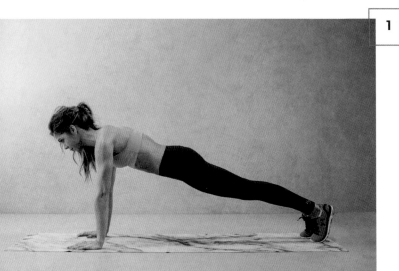

1

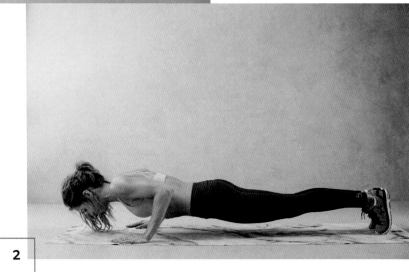

2

PUSH-UP

1. Begin in a plank position with your hands underneath your shoulders. Squeeze your core and glutes to keep your hips from sagging.

2. Bend your elbows and lower your chest until it almost touches the floor, then push yourself back up again. If this is too challenging, bend your knees to the floor.

TRICEP DIP

1. Sit on a bench (step or chair), position your hands shoulder-width apart and hold on to the edge.

2. Slide your bum off the edge so that your arms are fully extended, holding your body up, with your legs extended. If this is too challenging, bend your knees at a 90-degree angle.

3. From here, gently lower yourself by bending your elbows to about 90-degrees, ensuring you keep the elbows as close to your body as possible throughout the movement.

4. Using your arms, push up from here, squeezing your triceps at the top.

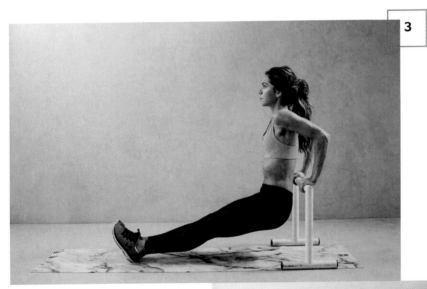

3

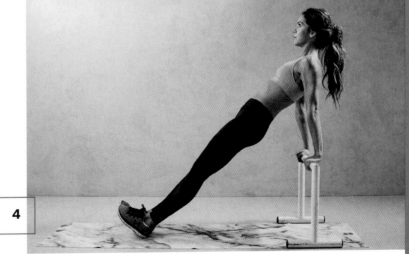

4

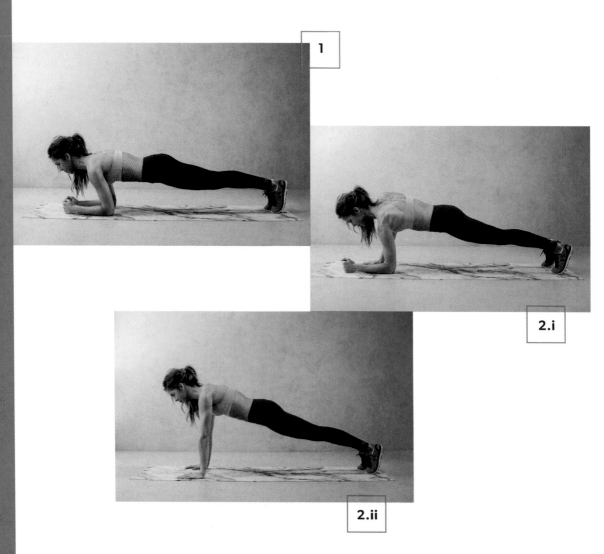

1

2.i

2.ii

PLANK TO PUSH-UP

1. Start in the same position as you would for a plank, with your body supported by the balls of your feet and your forearms.

2. Push yourself up onto your right hand and then immediately onto your left hand. Ensure that you squeeze your core and glutes to stop your body from swaying.

3. Return to the plank position by releasing your right hand and lowering onto your forearm, before doing the same with your left hand.

PUSH-UP WITH ROTATION

1. Get into a push-up position on the balls of your feet with your hands underneath your shoulders.

2. Do one push-up and as you come up, shift your weight on the right side of your body and twist your body to the left, bringing your left arm up towards the ceiling, to form a side plank.

3. Lower the arm back to the floor for another push-up and then twist to the other side.

4. Repeat the series, alternating each side, for the entire set of reps.

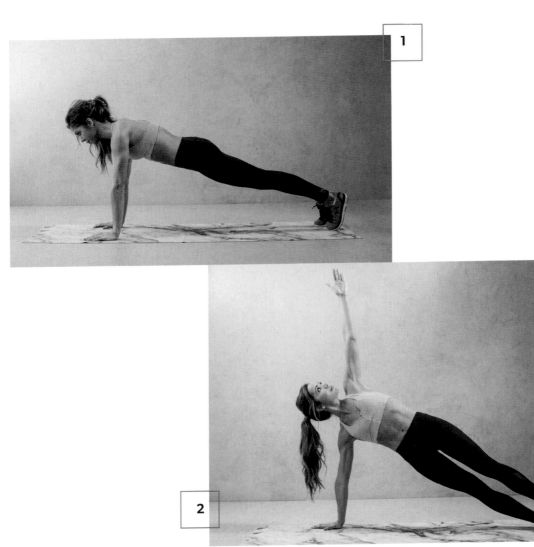

1

2

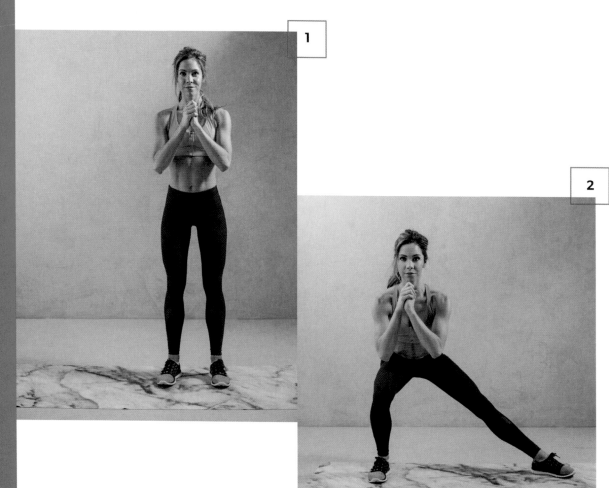

1

2

SIDE LUNGE

1. Stand straight with your feet shoulder-width apart, chest up, shoulders back and core tight. Your knees should have a soft bend. Hold your hands together as per the photo above.

2. Staying low, take a lateral step to the right. Extend your left leg so it is straight and shift your weight to the right, flexing your knee into a side lunge.

3. Pause at the bottom of the motion, and then extend through the working leg to return to a standing position, followed by a lunge to the opposite side. Alternate between each leg throughout the set.

FORWARD LUNGE

1. Stand straight with your feet shoulder-width apart, chest up, shoulders back and core tight. Your knees should have a soft bend and your hands held together.

2. Take a step forward with one foot and lower yourself to a point in which your rear knee almost touches the floor, maintaining your body's upright posture. Your front knee should have a 90-degree bend and be in line with, but just behind, your toes.

3. From the bottom position, push back up from your forward foot, bringing it back beside the other.

4. Repeat on the opposite side and alternate between each leg for the required number of repetitions.

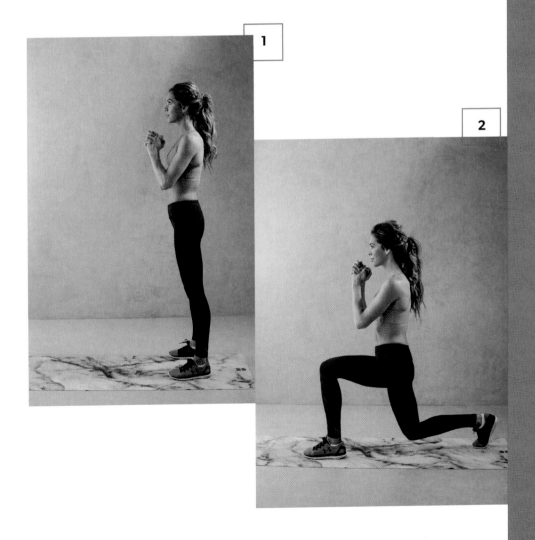

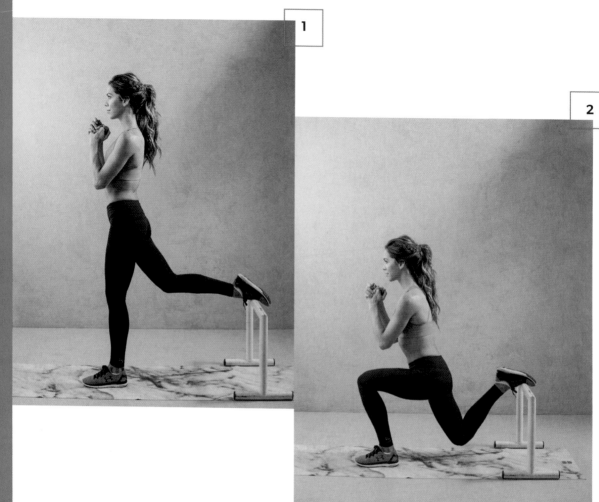

1

2

BULGARIAN SPLIT SQUAT

1. Stand in front of a step, at a distance comfortable for you to reach one leg back and rest your foot on top of the step. Clasp your hands together.

2. Bend your elevated leg at the knee, and slowly lower yourself towards the ground so that your knee comes close to the floor. The leading foot, which is on the floor, should be in line with your knee.

3. From here, push through your heel back to your starting position. Complete the required number of reps on one leg before moving on to the other leg.

SQUAT

1. Stand with your feet shoulder-width apart, chest up, shoulders back and core tight. Your knees should have a soft bend and your hands should be clasped together.

2. Start by flexing your knees and hips and then sit back into a squat until your hips are below your knees (if your mobility allows).

3. At the bottom of the squat, explode back up to a standing position, driving through heels.

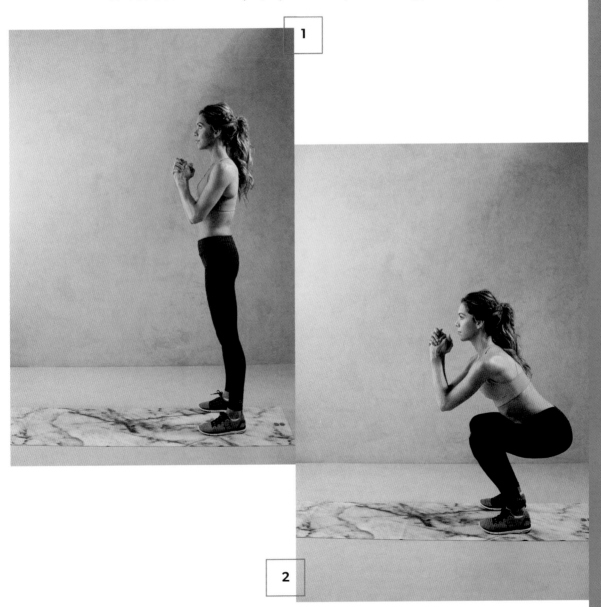

1

2

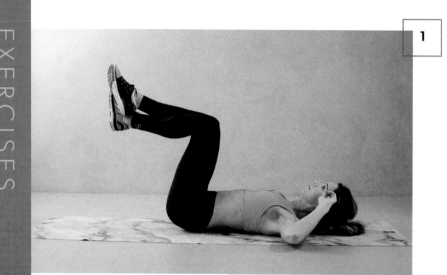

1

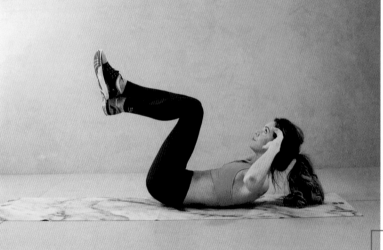

2

AB CRUNCH

1. Lie on the floor with your feet and knees off the floor and your knees at a 90-degree angle. Place your fingertips by the sides of your head.

2. Squeeze your core and raise your body up towards your knees, lifting your shoulders off the floor. Keep your head looking forward being careful not to strain your neck by pulling your neck forward or placing your chin on your chest.

3. Hold at the top for a moment, squeeze and slowly roll back down to the starting position.

FLUTTER KICK

1. Lie on your back with your legs straight and your arms extended above your head.

2. Lift your heels off the floor and rapidly kick your feet up and down in a quick, scissor-like motion.

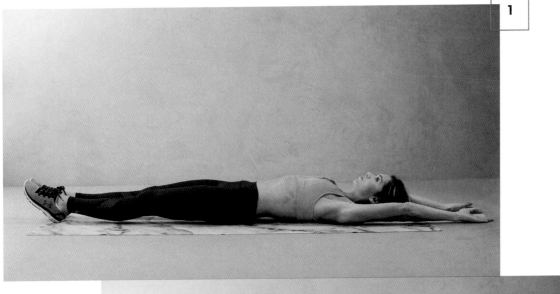

1

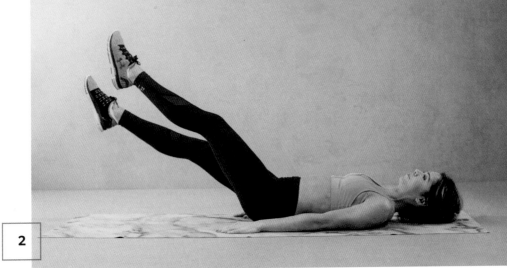

2

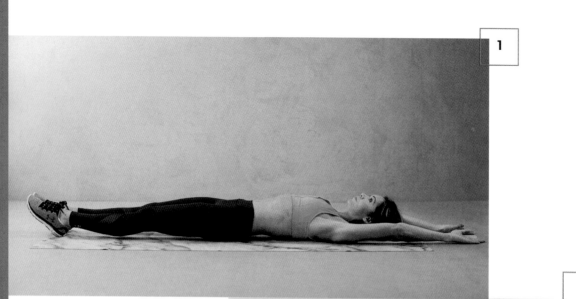

1

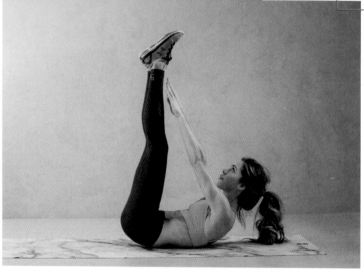

2

V-UP

1. Lie flat on the floor on your back with your arms and legs outstretched.

2. Squeeze your core and in one movement lift your legs up and raise your upper body up off the floor to touch your toes.

3. Slowly lower your body back down to the starting position.

MOUNTAIN CLIMBER

1. To begin, start in a push-up position with your hands shoulder-width apart on the floor. Your legs should be extended out behind you.

2. Bend one knee and bring it in towards your chest. Extend it back to the starting position and quickly repeat the same movement with the opposite leg.

3. Repeat in an alternating fashion for the required time or repetitions.

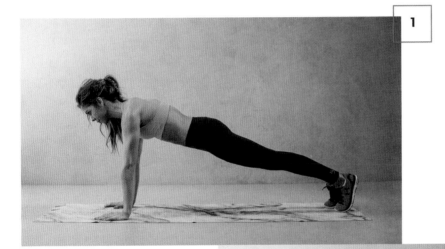

1

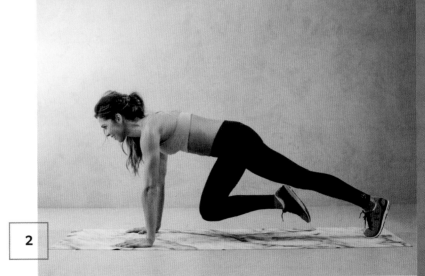

2

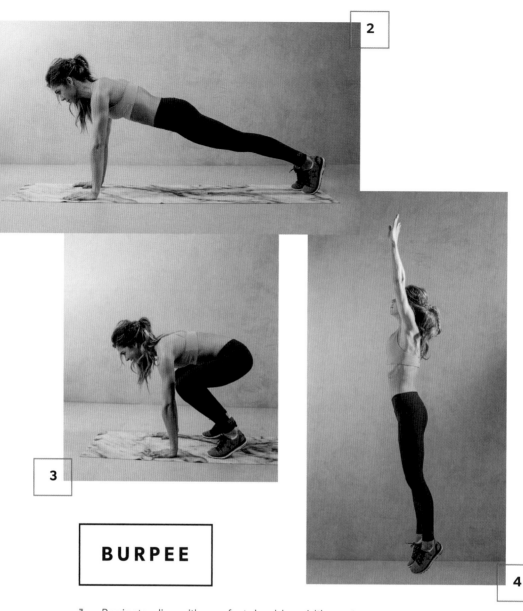

BURPEE

1. Begin standing with your feet shoulder-width apart.

2. Jump down into a plank position with your feet extended.

3. From here, jump your feet back towards your hands so that your knees are bent and your feet are under your hips.

4. Explosively jump into the air, reaching your arms straight overhead and land back in a standing position.

TUCK JUMP

1. Begin with your feet shoulder-width apart, chest up, shoulders back and core tight. Your knees should have a soft bend.

2. Quickly lower down into a quarter squat and jump up as high as you can, driving your knees towards your chest.

3. Bend your knees to cushion your landing and continue straight into the next rep.

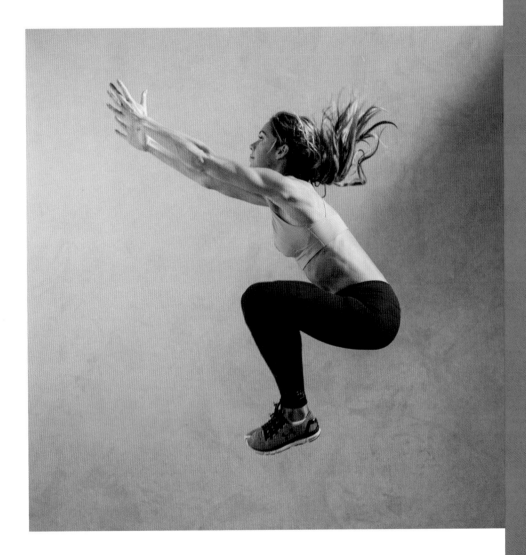

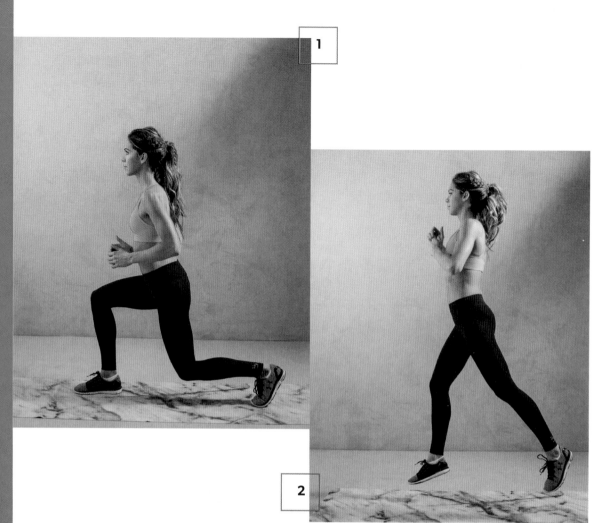

1

2

JUMP LUNGE

1. Stand with one foot in front of the other in a lunge position, with your back straight, shoulders back and your knees bent at a 90-degree angle. Push your chest out and lower your rear knee towards the ground in a lunge while keeping your front shin as vertical as possible.

2. Push explosively off the ground, jumping and switching the position of your legs while in mid-air, landing into the lunge position with the opposite leg forward.

3. Repeat, switching legs on each jump.

JUMP SQUAT

1. Begin with your feet shoulder-width apart, chest up, shoulders back and core tight. Your knees should have a soft bend.

2. Come down to a squatting position and quickly jump up, extending your legs straight underneath you.

3. Land in a squat position and pause for a moment, then repeat the movement.

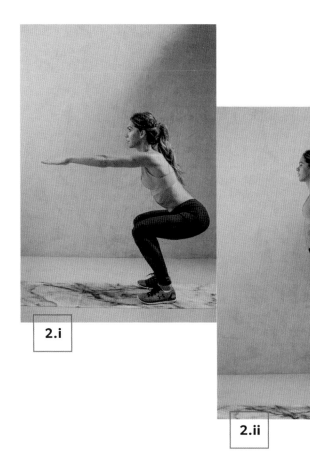

2.i

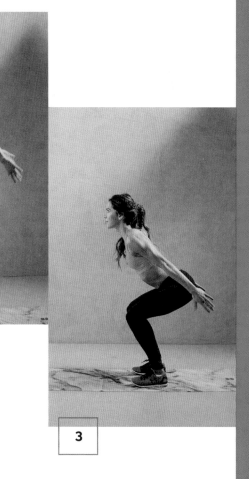

2.ii

3

THE PROTOCOLS

So here's where the fun begins. Now that you have an explanation of the exercises, it's time to pick one from each category (A,B,C, or D) and put them into a protocol.

Each protocol is basically a type of circuit. The reason I've given you lots of options to choose from is because I know how boring it can be when you follow the same old routine and workout day in, day out. This way you can try one type of circuit one day and another the next. You're less likely to get bored, your body will be challenged with new stimuli, and most importantly you're more likely to stick to it if you're enjoying it! This is my favourite way to train as I love challenging my body with new workouts. However, this is your body so you're in control of your workout. You choose the exercises, you choose the protocol, and you choose your goals!

AMRAP

As many rounds as possible (AMRAP) involves completing as many rounds of a circuit as you can in a given time with minimal rest. I love this protocol as you can use your previous score as a target to beat – so it's you vs you and no one else.

Choose four exercises, one from each group (A, B, C and D), and perform ten reps of each to complete one circuit. Set the timer for ten minutes and repeat the entire circuit as many times as you can until the buzzer stops.

AMRAP EXAMPLE:
Set your timer for ten minutes and complete the circuit continuously until the timer stops.

1. 10 x push-ups
2. 10 x side lunges
3. 10 x mountain climbers
4. 10 x burpees

EMOTM

Every minute on the minute (EMOTM) is a really simple protocol that involves performing one exercise for a specific number of reps, every minute for a select number of minutes. For every workout, use a timer and start each set at the beginning of every minute. Once you've completed the reps, rest for a couple of seconds until the next minute. The quicker you get through the reps, the more rest you will have before the next set starts. For this protocol, do ten reps of one exercise from group D, every minute for ten minutes.

EMOTM EXAMPLE:
Complete ten burpees every minute on the minute, for ten minutes.

TIP

For single leg exercises,
the number of repetitions
is for each leg, e.g. ten reps
of side lunges means ten
on each side.

TABATA

Tabata training was designed by Japanese scientist Dr Izumi Tabata and a team of researchers from the National Institute of Fitness and Sports in Tokyo. Don't be fooled by the length of this workout – it's a lot harder than it sounds. Choose an exercise and perform alternating intervals of twenty seconds of all-out effort with ten seconds of rest. Continue to repeat the same move for eight rounds, resulting in a total of four minutes.

I usually throw this circuit in at the end of my usual workout in the gym or use it as a super-quick workout before work in the morning. If you have more time and wish to push yourself a little harder, do four Tabata workouts with one exercise from each of the groups (A, B, C and D) so your entire workout will be sixteen minutes in total.

TABATA EXAMPLE:

- ROUND 1: 20s push-ups, 10s rest
- ROUND 2: 20s push-ups, 10s rest
- ROUND 3: 20s push-ups, 10s rest
- ROUND 4: 20s push-ups, 10s rest
- ROUND 5: 20s push-ups, 10s rest
- ROUND 6: 20s push-ups, 10s rest
- ROUND 7: 20s push-ups, 10s rest
- ROUND 8: 20s push-ups, 10s rest

COMPLEX

A complex is basically a series of exercises performed back-to-back in which the set number of reps is completed for each exercise before moving on to the next. This protocol is less complex than it sounds – it's actually the most basic of them all (but not any easier). Each workout consists of four exercises, one from each group (A ,B, C and D). Complete ten reps of each, then move on to the next without resting. Repeat the entire circuit for ten rounds, taking ten to twenty second breaks in between each round.

COMPLEX EXAMPLE:

- A.   10 x tricep dips
- B.   10 x Bulgarian split squats
- C.   10 x V-ups
- D.   10 x tuck jumps

10–20s rest after each round.
Repeat entire circuit x 10.

DESCENDING

The good news about this routine is that it gets easier as you go along. The bad news is that it starts out really difficult!

Choose four exercises, one from each group (A, B, C and D), and perform ten reps of each to complete the first step of the descending ladder. For the second set, complete nine reps of each exercise, and then for the third set complete eight reps . . . and so on, all the way down to the tenth set, which involves one rep of each exercise.

DESCENDING WORKOUT EXAMPLE:

- ROUND 1: 10 x plank to push-ups, 10 x squats, 10 x flutter kicks, 10 x jump lunges

- ROUND 2: 9 x plank to push-ups, 9 x squats, 9 x flutter kicks, 9 x jump lunges…

- ROUND 10: 1 x plank to push-up, 1 x squat, 1 x flutter kick, 1 x jump lunge

ASCENDING

This protocol starts with one rep of each exercise and works up, set by set, to ten reps of each exercise. So it gets harder as you approach the end!

Choose four exercises, one from each group (A, B, C and D), and perform one rep of each to complete the first step of the ascending ladder. For the second set, complete two reps of each exercise and then for the third set, complete three reps and so on for ten rounds.

ASCENDING WORKOUT EXAMPLE:

- ROUND 1: 1 x push-up with rotation, 1 x side lunge, 1 x sit-up , 1 x burpee

- ROUND 2: 2 x push-ups with rotation, 2 x side lunges, 2 x sit-ups, 2 x burpees…

- ROUND 10: 10 x push-ups with rotation, 10 x side lunges, 10 x sit-ups, 10 x burpees

GLOSSARY

AGAVE NECTAR

This all-natural sweetener is often championed as a healthy alternative to sugar due to its low glycemic index. For this reason, agave is sometimes favoured by diabetics. However, it still does contain sugar in the form of fructose. So if you do wish to include it in your diet, keep it to a minimum as you would any other sugar or sugar-alternative. For vegans, it is a popular substitute for honey, which is why you will see it in many of my recipes!

ALZHEIMER'S DISEASE

Alzheimer's disease is a type of dementia. The word dementia describes a set of symptoms that can include memory loss, changes in behaviour, difficulty concentrating and thinking. Alzheimer's disease is caused by a combination of genetic, lifestyle and environmental factors that affect the brain over time. According to a growing body of evidence, risk factors for vascular disease – including high blood pressure and high cholesterol – are also risk factors for Alzheimer's.

AMINO ACIDS

Amino acids are the building blocks of protein. They are responsible for manufacturing and repairing cells. There are twenty-one amino acids in total, some of which are essential and some non-essential. Essential amino acids cannot be made by the body and must be obtained through our diet, they are: isoleucine, leucine, lysine, methionine, phenylalanine, threonine, tryptophan and valine.

ANTIOXIDANTS

Antioxidants are molecules that prevent cell damage caused by other, unstable molecules in the body known as 'free radicals'. Antioxidants interact with and neutralise free radicals, thus preventing them from causing damage. The body can make some of the antioxidants it uses; however, we can also obtain them through our diet. Examples of dietary antioxidants include beta-carotene and vitamins A, C and E.

ATHEROSCLEROSIS

Atherosclerosis is a disease where plaque builds up inside the arteries. Over time, this causes the narrowing of the vessel lumen, which limits the flow of oxygen-rich blood to the organs, such as the heart and the brain. This can lead to health problems including heart attack and stroke.

CALORIE

A calorie is defined as the amount of energy required to raise the temperature of 1 gram of water by 1 degree Celsius. However, in simple terms, it is the unit of energy of food. The important word to take away from this definition is ENERGY. Calories are energy that fuel our bodies. Different macronutrients (carbohydrates, fats and proteins) provide a different amount of calories per gram.

CARDIOVASCULAR DISEASE

Cardiovascular disease (CVD) is an umbrella term for all diseases of the heart and blood vessels, including coronary heart disease, stroke and high blood pressure.

CHOLESTEROL

Cholesterol is a fatty substance made in the body by the liver, but also found in some foods. It is essential for the production of vitamin D, bile salts and hormones. However, having excessively high levels of cholesterol in your blood can be a risk factor for health conditions, such as heart disease and stroke. There are two main types of cholesterol in the bloodstream: high-density lipoprotein (HDL) or 'good cholesterol' and low-density lipoprotein (LDL), known as 'bad cholesterol'. The amount of cholesterol in the blood – both HDL and LDL – can be measured with a blood test.

COCONUT SUGAR

Coconut sugar, or coconut

blossom, is extracted from the sap of the coconut palm tree. You can buy it in a syrup or as a golden crystallised sugar. Coconut sugar has a low glycemic index and contains less fructose than white sugar. I'm a big fan of it in baking as it offers a similar taste to brown sugar making it a great lower-sugar alternative.

COELIAC DISEASE

Coeliac disease is an autoimmune condition where the body's defence system mistakes gluten as a threat and fights back by producing antibodies to fight it. This reaction damages the surface of the small bowel, interfering with the body's ability to absorb nutrients from food and causing symptoms, such as diarrhoea, abdominal pain and weight loss.

DETOX

The term 'detox' means detoxification which is a normal bodily process carried out by the liver to remove toxic substances from the body, such as ammonia, waste products, drugs and alcohol. This word is often misused as a buzzword for 'cleansing' or 'flushing' out toxins from our body with the use of supplements or foods.

DIABETES

Diabetes is a condition where the body does not make enough insulin or cannot use insulin properly. This causes blood sugar levels to become too high which, if left untreated, can lead to serious health complications including heart disease, blindness and kidney failure.

FREE RADICALS

Free radicals are unstable molecules which can cause cell damage. They may be formed naturally in the body but also from the environment as a result of diet, stress, cigarette smoke, UV radiation, toxins and pollutants. Under normal conditions the body can regulate free radicals; however, an excessive build-up of free radicals can cause them to interact with, and damage, cells in the body. This process, known as oxidative stress, has b een linked to many diseases, such as cancer, Alzheimer's and the ageing process.

GLUTEN

Gluten is a family of proteins found in certain grains, such as wheat, rye and barley. Gluten gives elasticity, strength and the ability to 'hold' food products together, such as bread, pizza and pastries.

GLUTEN-FREE OATS

The concept of gluten-free oats can be confusing as oats do not naturally contain gluten. However, they do contain a similar protein called avenin, to which about 5 per cent of coeliacs are intolerant. As most brands process their oats in facilities that also process other gluten-containing grains, such as wheat, barley and rye, they can also be contaminated with gluten. So if you are very intolerant to gluten, make sure you buy the certified gluten-free versions.

GRASS-FED MEAT

Grass-fed meat simply means the animal was raised on grass, not grain. Animals are often fed grain as it is more calorie-dense than grass, so it fattens them up faster. However, the beef is not as good quality as grass-fed. Grass-fed beef has better fat quality. Specifically, it has significantly more anti-inflammatory Omega 3 fats and significantly fewer inflammatory Omega 6 fats. Another reason grass-fed meat trumps grain-fed is that it contains considerably more antioxidants, vitamins and minerals – so if you can afford to spend a little extra, opt for grass-fed.

GUT MICROBIOME

The gut microbiome, also known as the gut flora, is the collective term for all the bacteria and other microorganisms that live in the human gut. The healthy bacteria in our gut are important for digestion, a strong immune system and making certain vitamins.

HIIT

High-Intensity Interval Training (HIIT) describes any workout that alternates between intervals of max effort and intervals of low-intensity activity or rest.

HONEY

Honey is not only useful for sweetening your morning porridge, it also has health benefits, such as antibacterial and antiviral activity. The medicinal properties of honey, particularly Manuka, means that you can

now find it in many wound care dressings used in current medical practice. Honey is still high in sugar, but it is packed full of important nutrients and antioxidants and so makes a sensible switch from refined white table sugar. When choosing honey, try to opt for raw or Manuka honeys which have the most enzymes and nutrients.

INSULIN

Insulin is a hormone released by the pancreas, a gland that sits underneath the stomach, in response to glucose in the bloodstream. Once insulin is in the blood, it shuttles glucose into the cells of the body to use as energy.

IRRITABLE BOWEL SYNDROME

Irritable Bowel Syndrome (IBS) is a very common digestive condition. IBS is an illness that has no known cause, no physical abnormality, and no diagnostic test. Symptoms are variable and include abdominal pain, bloating and bouts of diarrhoea and/or constipation.

LISS

LISS stands for Low-Intensity Sustained State, and it is a form of low-intensity exercise. This type of cardiovascular training typically involves working for a longer period of time, at a target heart rate of about 45–60 per cent of your maximum. An example of this would be walking on the treadmill or swimming.

MACRONUTRIENTS

Macronutrients, often referred to as 'macros', consist of three fundamental food groups: protein, carbohydrates and fats. These nutrients provide energy to the body in the form of calories.

METABOLISM

Metabolism is a term used to describe all of the chemical processes that go on inside the body to keep you alive, such as breathing, muscle contraction and digestion. All these processes require energy and the minimum amount of energy that your body uses to carry out these normal bodily functions is called the basal metabolic rate (BMR).

MICRONUTRIENTS

Micronutrients include vitamins and minerals. They are termed 'micro' as we only need them in small amounts. Unlike macronutrients, they do not provide energy but they are essential to our health as they enable the chemical reactions in our body to occur. Micronutrients are found in all whole foods so if you're eating a variety of fruit, vegetables, meat and fish then you probably don't need to worry about being deficient.

NUT BUTTER

Peanut, cashew, almond, hazelnut, macadamia nut butter – all taste wonderful and make great additions to baking and snacks, but they're also high in protein and healthy fats. One thing to keep in mind is that they are highly calorific, so if you're watching your weight, try your best to stop at one spoon.

ORGANIC

The word 'organic' is defined by law and anything labelled as such must meet this strict set of standards which are set by the Soil Association in the UK. The standards restrict the use of artificial chemical fertilisers and pesticides, prohibit Genetically Modified (GM) crops and ingredients, and ban the use of irradiation industrial solvents or chemical food additives. Simply put, organic means the product is 100 per cent naturally grown and minimally processed. Organic is more expensive than non-organic produce but choosing organic whenever you can afford to is a no-brainer. Pesticides are poisons designed to kill organisms, so why eat them if you can choose not to?

PALEO

The concept of the paleo diet is to basically eat like our ancestors from the paleolithic period which means to eat only foods you can hunt or find. In short, if a caveman couldn't eat it then neither can you! Following this diet means you eliminate all processed food from your diet and instead load up on organic meats, fish, nuts and vegetables. The paleo diet also excludes dairy as, beyond drinking breast milk during infancy, no other form of dairy was consumed in the paleolithic era.

PHYTOCHEMICALS

Phytochemicals are a large group of plant-derived compounds that are believed to confer health benefits to the body. They can be found in foods, such as fruit, vegetables, beans, cocoa and plant-based beverages, such as tea and wine. As they are not considered 'essential' to the diet, they do not fall into the same bracket as vitamins – but are still very good for you!

PREBIOTIC

Prebiotics are non-digestible fibres that allow healthy gut bacteria to survive and thrive. Foods rich in prebiotics include bananas, oats, legumes and fibrous vegetables.

PROBIOTIC

Probiotics are good bacteria, lactobacillus and bifidobacteria, that colonise our gut. Probiotics help to support our gut health through the digestion of food, absorption of nutrients, production of vitamins and protection of the gut lining against pathogenic strains of bacteria. Some foods naturally contain probiotics including natural yogurt, cottage cheese, sauerkraut and tempeh.

PROTEIN POWDER

This is essentially a powdered version of their whole food counterpart. Many people seem to worry that they're 'unnatural' or processed foods. As they are a powder, they are a byproduct of food so yes they are processed to some extent – but it doesn't make them any less real or 'bad' for you. The most widely available protein powder on the

market is whey protein, which is a dairy protein. It has a complete amino acid profile which means that it contains all the essential amino acids (i.e. the one's we can't make in the body ourselves). However, as the health and fitness industry expands you can now buy an array of protein powders that are non-dairy or vegan, such as hemp, brown rice and pea protein.

QUARK

Quark is a dairy product, similar to Greek yogurt and sour cream. Yet it's not quite cheese and not quite yogurt. In terms of nutrition, Quark is a great food to include in your diet. It's higher in protein than most other dairy products (it has about double the amount of protein in Greek yogurt) and contains trace amounts of natural sugar. It's also naturally low in fat, which means it tends to be low in calories too. This makes it a great alternative to cream cheese or cream when baking desserts, such as cheesecake or carrot cake. I also use it in savoury dishes instead of crème fraîche to cool down hot chillis or to add a creamy texture to sauces.

STEVIA

Stevia is a concentrated extract from the leaves of the stevia plant. It can be bought as a fine white powder or a liquid. It's super-sweet and can have a bit of an aftertaste, so you really don't need much of it. One of the biggest benefits of this sweetener is that it is 100 per cent calorie-free, so it has no effect on blood sugar, which is good news for anyone who has issues with

blood sugar control. I add it to coffee, oatmeal and smoothies.

SUPERFOOD

Superfoods are nutrient-dense foods that are especially rich in vitamins, minerals or antioxidants. The word 'superfood' is often over-used, and arguably misused, within the food industry as a marketing ploy to sell more of a particular product. There is no official definition of the word and the EU has banned health claims on packaging unless supported by scientific evidence. Foods that have been given the superfood status in recent years include those rich in antioxidants and omega 3 fatty acids.

TAHINI

Tahini is sort of like peanut butter, except it's made from sesame seeds. It's much saltier than a nut butter but it has a lovely silky consistency which makes the creamiest dressings and dips. It's also packed full of healthy polyunsaturated fats so it's great for your heart too.

TAMARI

Tamari is similar to soy sauce, in terms of origin and taste – they are both byproducts of fermented soya beans. The main difference between the two is the presence of wheat. In my recipes, you can use them interchangeably depending on your dietary requirements (or whatever is easiest to source).

REFERENCES

PROTEINS

• British Nutrition Foundation, (2016). *Nutrition Requirements*. [PDF] Available at: www.nutrition.org.uk/attachments/article/234/Nutrition%20Requirements_Revised%20Oct%202016.pdf [Accessed 30 January 2017].
• British Nutrition Foundation, (2012). *Protein*. [online] Available at: www.nutrition.org.uk/nutritionscience/nutrients-food-and-ingredients/protein.html [Accessed 30 January 2017].
• Cataldo, D, and Blair, M (2015). Protein Intake for Optimal Muscle Maintenance. *American College of Sports Medicine* [PDF] Available at: www.acsm.org/docs/default-source/brochures/protein-intake-for-optimal-muscle-maintenance.pdf [Accessed 30 January 2017].
• Paddon-Jones, D., Westman, E., Mattes, R., Wolfe, R., et al. (2008). Protein, weight man-agement, and satiety. *The American Journal of Clinical Nutrition*, Volume 87 (5) 1558S-1561S.

CARBOHYDRATES

• Mergenthaler, P., Lindauer, U., Dienel, G., Meisel, A. (2013). Sugar for the brain: the role of glucose in physiological and pathological brain function. *Trends Neurosci.*, Volume 36 (10), pp. 587–597.

FIBRE

• Brown, L., Rosner, B., Willett, W., Sacks, F. (1999). Cholesterol-lowering effects of dietary fiber: a meta-analysis. *The American Journal of Clinical Nutrition*, Volume 69 (1), pp. 30–42.
• Crowe, F., Balkwill, A., Cairns, B., Appleby, P., et al. (2014). Source of dietary fibre and di-verticular disease incidence: a prospective study of UK women. *Gut* 63:1450-1456.
• Howarth, N.C., Saltzman E., Roberts, S.B., (2001). Dietary fiber and weight regulation. *Nutrition Reviews*, Volume 59 (5), pp. 129–139.
• Scientific Advisory Committee on Nutrition,(2015). Carbohydrates and Health. *SACN: reports and position statements*. Norwich: TSO (The Stationery Office) [PDF] Available at: www.gov.uk/government/uploads/system/uploads/attachment_data/file/445503/SACN_Carbohydrates_and_Health.pdf [Accessed 30th January 2017].
• Threapleton, D., Greenwood, D., Evans, C., Cleghorn, et al. (2013). Dietary fibre intake and risk of cardiovascular disease: systematic review and meta-analysis. *BMJ* ;347:f6879.

FATS

• British Nutrition Foundation, (2016) *Good fats and bad fats explained*. [online] Available at: www.nutrition.org.uk/healthyliving/basics/fats.html [Accessed 30 January 2017].
• DiNicolantonio, J., Lucan, S., O'Keefe, J. (2016). The Evidence for Saturated Fat and for Sugar Related to Coronary Heart Disease. *Progress in Cardiovascular Diseases*, Volume 58 (5), pp. 464–472.
• Kris-Etherton, P. (1999). Monounsaturated Fatty Acids and Risk of Cardiovascular Disease. *Circulation*, Volume 100 (11), pp. 1253–1258.
• Millán J, Pintó X, Muñoz A, et al. Lipoprotein ratios: Physiological significance and clinical usefulness in cardiovascular prevention (2009) *Vascular Health and Risk Management, Vol 5:*757-765.
• Patterson, E., Wall, R., Fitzgerald, G., Ross, R., Stanton, C. (2012). Health Implications of High Dietary Omega-6 Polyunsaturated Fatty Acids. *Journal of Nutrition and Metabolism, Vol. 2012*.

NUTRITION MYTHS

• Coeliac UK, (2016). *Coeliac disease key facts and stats 2016* [PDF] Available at: www.coeliac.org.uk/document-library/25-key-facts-and-stats/?return=/about-us/media-centre/ [Accessed 30 January 2017].
• Granata, G., and Brandon, L. (2014). The Thermic Effect of Food and Obesity: Discrepant Results and Methodological Variations. *Nutrition Reviews*, Volume 60 (8), pp. 223–233.
• Rippe, J., and Angelopoulos, T. (2015). Sugars and Health Controversies: What Does the Science Say? *Advances in Nutrition*, Vol. 6: 493S-503S.

CALORIES

• Westerterp, K. (2004). Diet induced thermogenesis. *Nutrition & Metabolism*, 18;1(1):5.
• Westman EC, Mavropoulos J, Yancy WS, Vlek JS (2003) A review of low-carbohydrate ketogenic diets. *Current Atherosclerosis Reports* 2003, 5:476–483[PDF] Available at: www.omega3galil.com/wp-content/uploads/2013/10/A-Review-of-Low-carbohydrate.pdf [Accessed 30 January 2017].

THE HEART+BLOOD VESSELS

• Aller, R., Antonio de Luis, D., Izaola, O., La Calle, F., et al (2004). Effect of soluble fiber intake in lipid and glucose levels in healthy subjects : a randomized clinical trial. *Diabetes Research and Clinical Practice*, Volume 65 (1), pp. 7–11.

• British Heart Foundation, (2017). *CVD Statistics – BHF UK Factsheet*. [online] Available at: www.bhf.org.uk/research/heart-statistics [Accessed 30 January 2017].

• Borghouts, L., Keizer, H. (2000). Exercise and insulin sensitivity: a review. *Int J Sports Med*.;21(1):1-12. Brown, L., Rosner, B., Willett, W., Sacks, F. (1999).

• Cholesterol-lowering effects of dietary fiber: a meta-analysis. *The American Journal of Clinical Nutrition*, Volume 69 (1), pp. 30–42.

• Consensus Action on Salt & Health (2010) *Salt and cardiovascular disease*. [online] Available at: www.actiononsalt.org.uk/salthealth/factsheets/stroke/ [Accessed 30 January 2017].

• Eilat-Adar, S., Sinai, T., Yosefy, C., Henkin, T. (2013). Nutritional Recommendations for Cardiovascular Disease Prevention. *Nutrients*, vol 5, 3646-3683.

• Kris-Etherton, P., Harris, W., Appel, L. (2002). Fish Consumption, Fish Oil, Omega-3 Fatty Acids, and Cardiovascular Disease. *Circulation*, 106:2747-2757 [PDF] Available at: circ.ahajournals.org/content/106/21/2747 [Accessed 30 January 2017].

• Lunn, J., Buttriss, J. (2007). Carbohydrates and dietary fibre. *Nutrition Bulletin*, 32: 21–64.

• Mann, S., Beedie, C., Jimenez, A. (2014). Differential Effects of Aerobic Exercise, Resistance Training and Combined Exercise Modalities on Cholesterol and the Lipid Profile: Review, Synthesis and Recommendations. *Sports Medicine*, Volume 44 (2), pp. 211–221.

• Threapleton, D., Greenwood, D., Evans, C., Cleghorn, C., et al. (2013). Dietary fibre intake and risk of cardiovascular disease: systematic review and meta-analysis, *BMJ; 347:f6879*

• Whelton, S., Chin, A., Xin, X., He, J., (2002). Effect of Aerobic Exercise on Blood Pressure: A Meta-Analysis of Randomized, Controlled Trials. *Annals of Internal Medicine*, Volume 136 (7), pp. 493–503.

THE BRAIN

• Bourre, J.-M. (2005). Dietary Omega-3 Fatty Acids and Psychiatry: Mood, Behaviour, Stress, Depression, Dementia and Ageing. *J Nutr Health Aging*, 9(1):31-8.

• Chang, C., Ke, D., Chen, J. (2009). Essential fatty acids and human brain. Acta Neurologica Taiwanica,Volume 18 (4), pp. 231–241.

• Foster, J., McVey Neufeld, K.-A. (2013). Gut-brain axis: how the microbiome influences anxiety and depression. *Trends in Neurosciences*, Volume 36 (5), pp. 305–312.

• Patterson, E., Wall, R., Fitzgerald, G., Ross, R., Stanton, C. (2012). Health Implications of High Dietary Omega-6 Polyunsaturated Fatty Acids. *Journal of Nutrition and Metabolism*, Vol. 2012.

• Steenbergen, L., Sellaro, R., van Hemert, S., Bosch, J., Colzato, L. (2015). A randomized controlled trial to test the effect of multispecies probiotics on cognitive reactivity to sad mood. *Brain Behavior and Immunity*, Volume 48, pp. 258–264.

THE DIGESTIVE SYSTEM

• Mayer, E., Craske, M., Naliboff, B. (2001). Depression, Anxiety, and the Gastrointestinal System. *The Journal of Clinical Psychiatry*, Vol 62 (8), pp. 28–36; discussion 37.

• NICE, (2008). *Irritable bowel syndrome in adults: diagnosis and management*. [online] Available at: www.nice.org.uk/guidance/cg61/chapter/introduction [Accessed 30 January 2017].

• Quigley, E. (2013). Gut Bacteria in Health and Disease. *Gastroenterology & Hepatology*, Volume 9 (9), pp. 560–569.

HAIR, SKIN + NAILS

• Balbás, G. M., Regaña, M. S., & Millet, P. U. (2011). Study on the use of omega-3 fatty acids as a therapeutic supplement in treatment of psoriasis. *Clinical, Cosmetic and Investigational Dermatology*, Vol. 4, 73–77.

• Cosgrove, M., Franco, O., Granger, S., Murray, P., Mayes, A. (2007). Dietary nutrient in-takes and skin-ageing appearance among middle-aged American women. *The American Journal of Clinical Nutrition*, [online] Volume 86 (4), pp. 1225–1231.

GLOSSARY

• Diplock, A., Charleux, J.-L., Grozier-Willi, G., Kok, F., Rice-Evans, C., et al(1998). Func-tional food science and defence against reactive oxidative species. *British Journal of Nutrition*, vol, 80 (1) S77-S112.

• Kivipelto, M., Helkala, E.-L., Laakso, M., Hänninen, T., et al. (2001). Midlife vascular risk factors and Alzheimer's disease in later life: longitudinal, population based study, *BMJ* ;322:1447.

• Lobo, V., Patil, A. Phatak, A., Chandra, N. (2010). Free radicals, antioxidants and functional foods: Impact on human health. *Pharmacognosy Reviews*, Volume 4 (8), pp. 118–126.

INDEX

ACKNOWLEDGEMENTS

I want to start by thanking the whole team at Yellow Kite for all the hard work, talent, and passion which went into creating this book. A special thanks to my publisher, Liz Gough, and editor, Tamsin English, for embracing my vision and believing in the message of The Food Medic.

To my literary agent, Carly Cook, who first spotted potential in The Food Medic and encouraged me to write this book. Thank you for your patience, guidance, and most of all, your friendship, throughout the process.

To my agency, Crown, but most importantly my agent, Jonny McWilliams, and my manager, Laura Johnson. Thank you for believing in me from the start and helping The Food Medic grow from strength to strength. We make a great team, and a great family.

Thank you to my incredible shoot team – Susan Bell, Nikki Dupin, Frankie Unsworth and Olivia Wardle. Together you created a book more beautiful than I could have ever asked for. I'm also incredibly grateful for the help and guidance from Adam Willis while on set.

To my mum: I simply can't put into words how grateful I am for all that you have done for me. You're the bravest, strongest woman I know. Without you, I wouldn't be where I am today. You held my hand through the hard times and nurtured me back to health and happiness with your ongoing love and support. To the rest of my family, my sisters: thank you for always being my number one supporters and best friends.

To my followers, or can I call you my friends? I don't count the numbers, but I can feel the magnitude of your support grow daily. Many of you have been there from the start when I was a young medical student, with big dreams and a small-time blog. Without you, I wouldn't have had the opportunity to write this book and share my passion. You inspire me to do great things.